JOYOUS DETOX

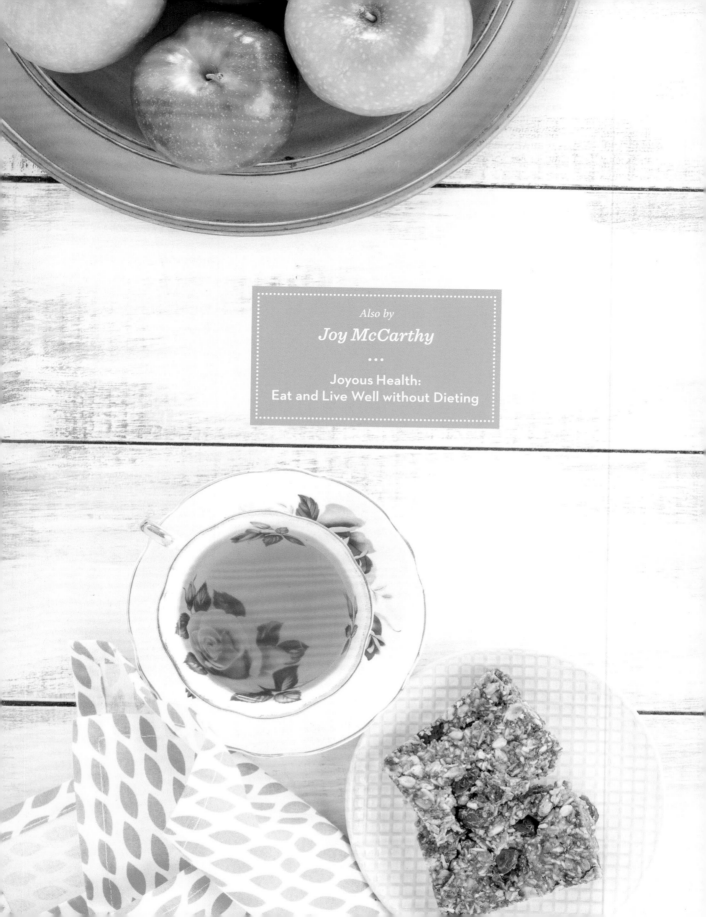

Also by

Joy McCarthy

• • •

Joyous Health:
Eat and Live Well without Dieting

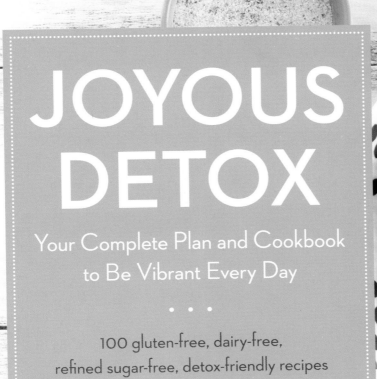

JOYOUS DETOX

Your Complete Plan and Cookbook to Be Vibrant Every Day

• • •

100 gluten-free, dairy-free,
refined sugar-free, detox-friendly recipes

JOY McCARTHY

PENGUIN

an imprint of Penguin Canada, a division of Penguin Random House Canada Limited

Canada • USA • UK • Ireland • Australia • New Zealand • India • South Africa • China

First published 2016

Photography by Chris Bodnar
Food and prop styling by Carol Dano

www.penguinrandomhouse.ca

LIBRARY AND ARCHIVES CANADA CATALOGUING IN PUBLICATION

McCarthy, Joy (Nutritionist), author
    Joyous detox : your complete plan and cookbook to be
vibrant every day / Joy McCarthy.

Includes index.
ISBN 978-0-14-319460-6 (paperback)
ISBN 978-0-14-319461-3 (electronic)

    1. Detoxification (Health). 2. Nutrition. 3. Cooking
(Natural foods). 4. Cookbooks. I. Title.

RA784.5.M34 2016   613.2   C2016-902530-6

Cover design by Jennifer Lum
Printed and bound in China

10 9 8 7 6 5 4 3 2 1

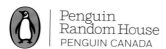

Penguin
Random House
PENGUIN CANADA

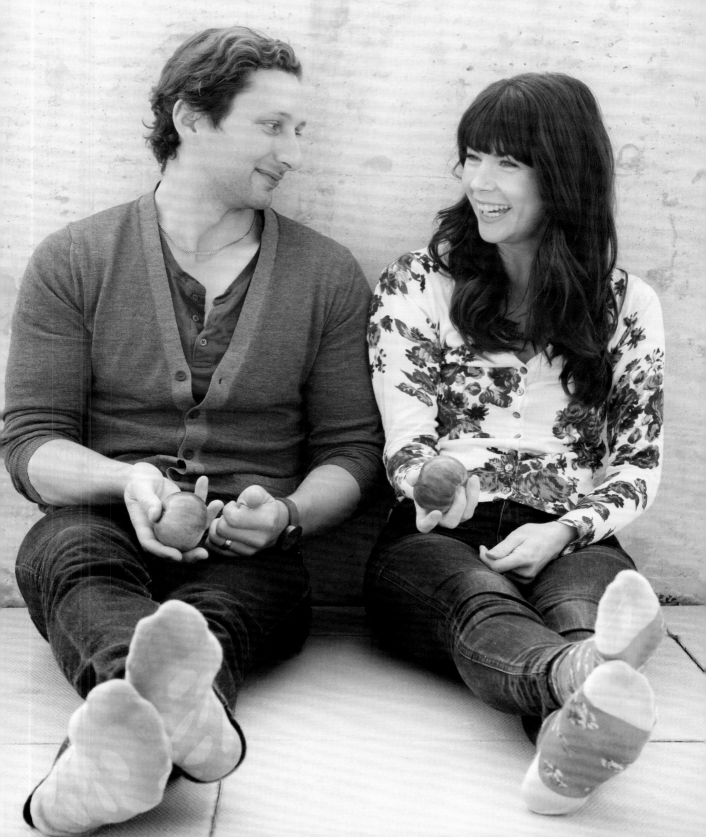

*This book is dedicated to my incredible husband,
my sunshine and my life partner, Walker Jordan, a.k.a. Walkman.*

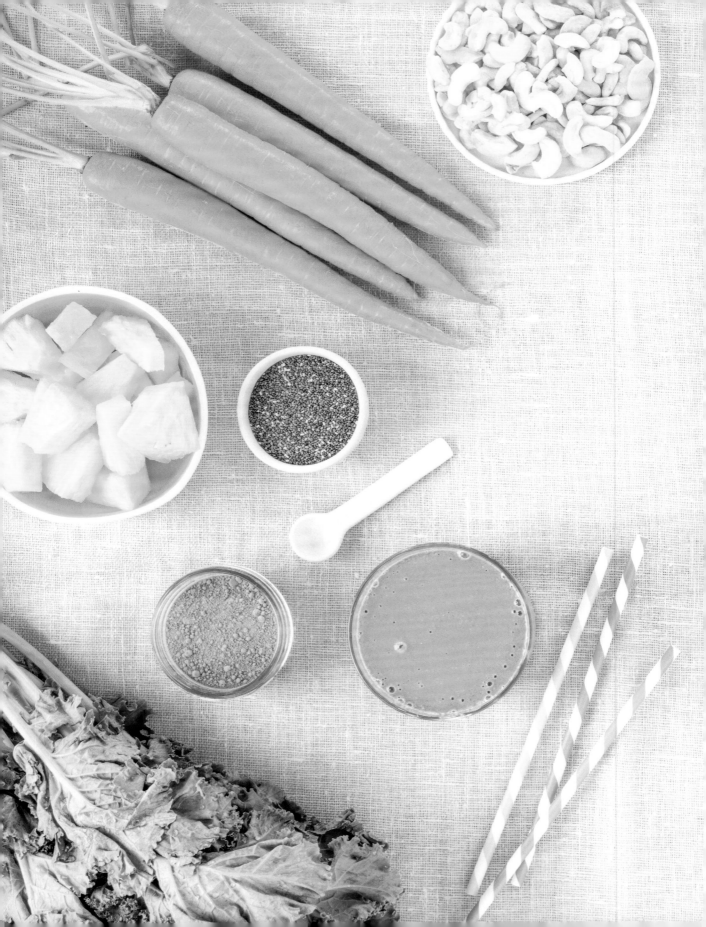

Contents

...

INTRODUCTION

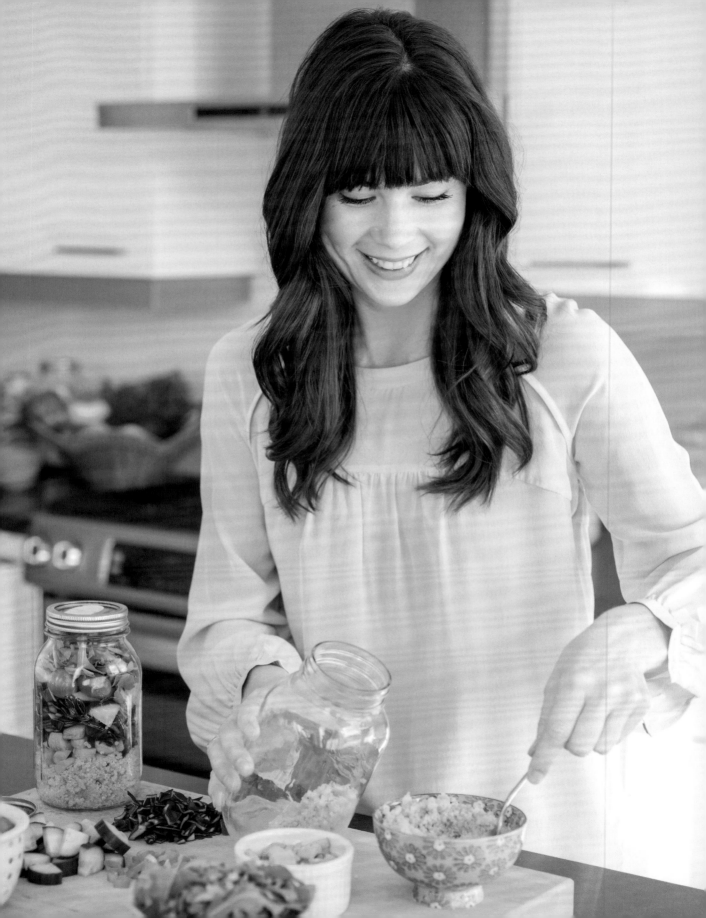

INTRODUCTION

There is no better time to start living healthy than now. You are the best person to take care of you! When you take care of you, you will have a joyful place to live for years to come.

—Joy McCarthy

MY STORY

In my twenties, I was completely addicted to sugar. I'm sure it didn't help that I was working at an advertising agency and my main client was a candy company. You can just imagine the number of freebies I received. Most of the time, I had hundreds of bags of chocolate-covered almonds and peanuts under my desk. Some might think this was heaven, but it was hell when I was trying my best *not* to indulge—not to become a downright ferocious sugar monster!

When I decided it was time to kick my sugar habit, I experimented with numerous cleanses and detoxes. Colon cleanses, juice fasts, raw food cleanses, liver detoxes—you name it, I have probably tried it. I kept trying things out well into the time I attended nutrition school. I thought, "How can I possibly recommend these cleanses and detoxes if I haven't tried them myself?" By experiencing so many different detoxes and cleanses myself, I've hopefully saved you from going down the same path—which more often than not was the path to the washroom!

That wasn't the only downside. More often than not, after just a few days I had little or no energy. That's not to say that none of these cleanses and detoxes had benefits, because some of them did. I just found it really difficult at times to stick with the prescribed programs, especially when the thought of downing another slimy green concoction would give me the dry heaves!

I started to realize that all those trendy—and sometimes severely restrictive—programs offered no benefit once I went back to my old ways of eating. And I had no choice but to go back to these old ways of eating because *most cleanses were simply not sustainable for health and well-being,* not to mention for giving me the energy to walk up a flight of stairs. And they certainly weren't reasonable if I wanted to maintain any sort of social life.

It was through my own experiences, my education and the journey that ultimately led me to become a certified nutritionist that I found my own effective detox, which I called the Joyous Detox.

Before settling on "Joyous Detox" as the title of this book, I was really drawn to "Everyday Detox." Let me tell you why. After trying to manage my diet by eating those 250-calorie frozen lunches and dinners in an effort to balance out my mid-afternoon candy fixes, I realized that the only way to kick my sweet tooth was to actually eat real food every day. What a concept—a healthy, whole, balanced diet that also included some natural sweeteners! The funny thing was, to most of my friends, this whole-food diet I was embarking on made it seem like I was living on a perpetual "detox." Yet I was feeling better than I had ever felt, and certainly better than I had ever felt doing those hard-core detoxes or cleanses. I had no more sugar cravings or energy crashes, my chronically bloated belly had deflated, and I looked and felt joyous. Everyone kept asking me what I was doing because I was glowing!

Some might call this book a detox book, but when you really delve into it, you'll find that it's an *everyday eating and living guide* to feeling joyous on the inside and glowing on the outside. I realized, though, that "Everyday Detox" was not a very snappy title, nor would most people have any clue what it meant, so I called my book *Joyous Detox*, because that's exactly how you will feel when you eat and live this way—joyous!

My promise to you is that you won't feel deprived working your way through my recipes. In fact, you'll feel completely the opposite. You'll feel nourished and inspired to live a healthy lifestyle.

This promise is based on the experiences of thousands of people who have participated in the popular Joyous 10-Day Detox, an online program that I offer on joyoushealth.com. Their involvement has given me incredible insight into what makes people commit to a program. It's not some quick-fix cleanse or detox—it's a lifestyle. Call it whatever your heart desires, but it works, and I'm so excited to take you on this journey with me. Here's what a few of my clients who've done the Joyous Detox have to say:

"I've just finished and I'm feeling awesome! My complexion has cleared, I've lost weight and strong cravings, I feel light and energized!" —*Karen*

"Since starting the Joyous Detox in February, I'm down 30 pounds, and I've kept it off since July!" —*Ashley*

"Finished my detox last Friday, and I'm so pleased with the results! I lost weight, my energy has soared, and I managed to stave off illness despite ALL of my co-workers being sick." —*Alison*

LET'S TALK DETOX!

Detoxification is the natural process by which the body removes toxic substances and chemicals. Eating a diet based on whole foods and emphasizing specific detox-friendly foods helps this process along. Giving your body a break from certain foods—including additives, sugar, bad fats and toxins—is also necessary for a successful detox. Of course you can also detox with the assistance of herbal teas, tinctures and supplements that help remove unwanted substances from your body. However, that's best done under the supervision of a certified natural healthcare practitioner.

There are hundreds of different detoxes on the market today, which might lead you to believe that we are all full of toxic sludge and chemical waste. Although this is a slight exaggeration, chemicals do accumulate in our bodies and cause a whole range of symptoms, from low energy and weight gain to skin problems, hormonal imbalance, immune dysfunction and even cancer. There is an absolute need to pay more attention to what we are feeding our bodies, what we are slathering on our skin and what we spray in the air and on ourselves.

While the human body is incredibly resilient, evolution has not (yet) modified our genes to effectively detoxify compounds that would otherwise kill insects, repel fire or stain-proof your couch. And that only scratches the surface of the number of chemical compounds your body comes into contact with every day. In fact, if we look at our food system, there are more than ten thousand chemicals in our food, from artificial sweeteners and flavouring to dyes, preservatives and more, according to the Center for Science in the Public Interest, and big corporations are coming up with new chemicals all the time. Believe me, these are not chemicals that enhance the nutrition of food for the benefit of our health. Beauty products are no better. Of the 82,000 ingredients used in personal care products, one in eight are industrial chemicals, among them carcinogens, pesticides, reproductive toxins and hormone disruptors. Pretty scary, isn't it?

Simply stated, our ancient biology cannot cope with our modern "chemical soup" environment. Our bodies don't have the ability to detoxify these substances effectively. In addition to the chemicals in and around us, our bodies also produce their own waste products through the process of cellular metabolism. In fact, even the gut bacteria that call your body home constantly release toxic waste products. Are you beginning to see why the Joyous Detox is so important?

I know this information might all feel a little overwhelming, but remember that having this knowledge is an incredibly powerful tool for us to take charge of our health. We can't rely on government intervention, so *we* must be responsible for the health and well-being of ourselves and our children.

THE POWER IS IN YOUR HANDS!

The ball is in your court. These chemicals are potentially hampering your health. What you eat and your lifestyle also affect how you are feeling and how healthy you are in this moment. You have the power to do something about it. Your choices are abundant every single second of every single day. You have the power to choose to clean your toilet bowl with toxic poisonous chemicals or to use an eco-friendly solution. You have the power to eat fast food or to put nourishing fruits and vegetables in your body.

So how does your body detoxify substances it deems harmful?

Your body has a network of systems and organs that help it to identify, neutralize and eliminate chemicals. Your liver, lungs, digestive system, lymphatic system, skin and urinary system work hard every single second of every day to transform chemicals into less threatening substances.

Your liver, being your master organ of detoxification, does most of the heavy lifting. The liver has a two-phase system for dealing with the toxins that make their way into your body. In phase one, known as oxidation, it uses specific enzymes on the toxin. Cytochrome P450 enzymes work their magic by making the toxin water-soluble, after which one of three things can happen.

1. The toxin gets sent to the sweat or urine to be eliminated through the skin or urinary system.
2. It gets sent into the bile to pass out through your feces when you have a bowel movement.
3. It gets converted to an intermediate compound that is sometimes more toxic than the original toxin.

This may sound like a smooth-running machine, but consider this. If you aren't drinking enough water and you are guzzling coffee all day (further dehydrating your body), your detox systems will struggle to eliminate toxins through your sweat and urine. Can you see how something as simple as being dehydrated can hamper natural detoxification?

Now, you may feel concerned about toxins that take the third option and get converted into something more harmful. Don't worry! In phase two of detoxification, known as conjugation, a whole host of chemical reactions occur in your liver that can neutralize harmful compounds created in phase one and convert them to a form that can be eliminated, as before, through your bile, sweat or urine.

Now that you know how your body detoxifies, you might be thinking, "Awesome! I don't need to change a thing because my body knows exactly what to do." Not so fast! Unfortunately, our bodies can become overburdened, stressed and tired. If this happens while you're eating the Standard American Diet, you're definitely not getting the nutrients you need for your natural detox systems to work effectively.

When the gas light comes on in your car, warning you that you need more gas, you pay attention, right? You know that if you don't fill up soon you'll run out of gas at a very inconvenient time. Not only that, you fuel up with the type of gas that your car requires. In other words, if you have a car that runs on gasoline, you don't fill it up with diesel or propane, because that would just be silly; the engine probably won't work very well either.

The same is true for the human body. If you put junk food—the wrong fuel—into your body, you will not function optimally. Sure, you'll get by on very nutrient-poor food, but at what cost? You might suffer for years from skin problems, low energy, weight gain, depression and brain fog without realizing that the food you fuel your body with is simply lacking the raw materials you need for energy, for vitality and to support the natural process of effective detoxification.

JOYOUS DETOX PLAN

The Joyous Detox plan is a healthy *and* enjoyable detox. You won't be depriving yourself or eating too few calories. Deprivation and calorie restriction can backfire by increasing your appetite hormones. Instead, as part of the Joyous Detox plan, you'll just take a break from specific foods and additives. (I'll discuss these in detail in chapter 1.) It is important to know what to avoid because navigating food labels can be a confusing and frustrating experience. But you'll soon be able to spot suspect food additives with ease!

Among the foods I suggest you avoid are refined sugar, dairy, gluten and coffee. If this sounds pretty much like your entire kitchen, not to worry, because I have included a whole chapter on all the delicious whole foods that I want you to enjoy every day. So be sure to read chapter 2, "Joyous Detox Superfoods." It's one of the most important chapters in the book. I say this because most detoxes and cleanses on the market today focus far too much on what to avoid, and I'm just not a fan of this approach. Every day we are bombarded with news about the latest chemical that is making us sick, what to avoid, what not to eat or what diet yields the best results. Being afraid of everything and thinking we are doing things wrong is a very negative way to live.

But here's the kicker: adding more good stuff means you have less room for the bad stuff. For example, if you fill your kitchen with plenty of nourishing foods, you simply have less space for those chips, cookies and packaged foods made in a lab. But don't worry, when following the Joyous Detox plan you will get to the point where even if you do have room for all that junk, you won't want it.

Detoxing goes beyond what you eat. So be sure to read chapter 3, "Detox Lifestyle Habits," because it includes amazing detox habits, including my favourite morning daily habit—dry skin brushing—along with plenty more life-altering detox habits to help your body better detoxify and help you feel vibrant and alive every day.

Since your Joyous Detox starts in the kitchen, turn to chapter 4 for tips to make over your kitchen, such as the importance of having a healthy snack shelf in your fridge and ditching canned foods. A healthy swap chart outlines common foods that you will want to ditch (some of them with sneaky ingredients) and what to replace them with so you don't miss your favourites. I will also review essential kitchen equipment and—for the keeners or gourmet cooks—some fancy kitchen gadgets to consider if your budget allows.

Creating a well-stocked kitchen is absolutely key to your success. You will learn what essentials to stock in your detox-friendly kitchen and how to store them. If you've got a kitchen packed with healthy and yummy foods, then you'll be far less likely to head to the grocery store for a bag of chips or a candy bar.

2-Day Reboot and 10-Day Joyous Detox plans

In chapter 5, I offer a 2-Day Reboot meal plan for after those weekends when you've overindulged and you need to hit the reset button. Keep in mind that this won't *undo* a weekend of beer and wings, but it *will* help you get back on the healthy eating track. There are also two 10-Day Detox meal plans for you to choose from, both Omnivore and Vegan (with vegetarian options), so you'll have plenty of choice.

Or you can simply work your way through my flavourful and detoxifying recipes as you see fit. The best part is that you get to eat delicious and nourishing food with an added benefit—my recipes incorporate ingredients that support the body's detoxification systems. These are recipes I personally eat every single day.

Before you jump in and decide which meal plan you will do, be sure to read all about pre-cleansing. This is especially important if you've never embarked on a healthy eating plan before. If you have been eating the Standard American Diet— SAD for short, and yes, it is indeed sad—you may experience a few pesky symptoms as you begin your Joyous Detox. But don't worry, they will be short-lived and you'll be feeling joyous in no time! Just refer to the Frequently Asked Questions on page 93 for tips on managing any symptoms.

I also give answers to questions such as what to do if you're craving sugar or if you have an event coming up where you know it will be tough to stay on track. I've got strategies galore! In fact, I can't think of a single situation you can't easily navigate and stay on track.

Last but not least is the most delicious part of the Joyous Detox—100 detoxifying, nourishing and tasty recipes in the final chapter.

Amazing benefits of the Joyous Detox plan

Here are just a few of the amazingly wonderful results you may experience in just a few days of following the Joyous Detox plan:

- increased energy and vitality
- vibrant glowing skin
- improved digestion
- weight loss
- reduced cravings
- reduced PMS or menopausal symptoms
- improved blood sugar balance
- positive mental outlook
- a feeling of empowerment

Before you jump into the detox, I strongly encourage you to read all the chapters. Together they contain the knowledge that is going to keep you motivated to continue on this path of wellness and vitality. **Knowledge is transformative and an essential part of the Joyous Detox experience.** That knowledge is the *why* behind doing this detox that will keep you feeling excited about all the positive changes you are about to experience. Remember those quotes I shared earlier? They were from people who had never done a detox before. If they can do it, so can you!

My hope is that you get to the point where you no longer see this plan as a "detox" but as a way of life—that eating this way will be what you want to do every single day. It's the Joyous Detox!

Please feel free to reach out to me through social media if you are feeling stuck or have a question:

- 🌐 joyoushealth.com
- 📘 Joyous Health.ca
- 🐦 @joyoushealth
- 📷 joyoushealth
- ▶ joyoushealth1
- 📌 Joyous Health
- 👤 Joyoushealth

If you're tweeting me or sharing your detox food photos through Instagram, be sure to use the hashtag #JoyousDetox.

If you follow me on Pinterest or on Instagram, you know I'm a big believer in manifesting what you desire, so be sure to check out some of my favourite affirmations on social media to keep handy on those days when you feel stuck or unmotivated. I've also included a special affirmation for you at the end of each chapter. I encourage you to read these aloud as many times as you need, and to reaffirm whenever you need some support to remind you of the positive path you have chosen.

Joyous Affirmation

I choose to be healthy and well
because I am the architect of my well-being.

1
FOODS TO AVOID

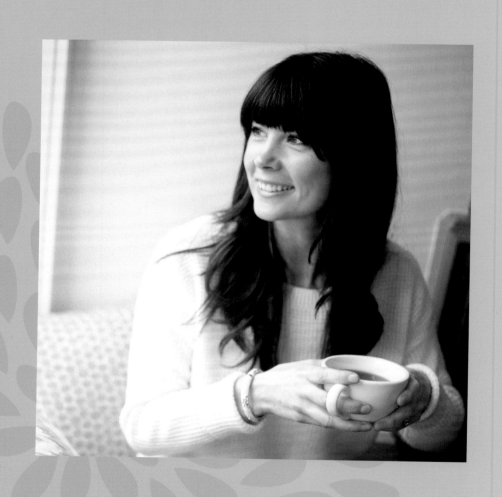

This is usually the topic people are most curious about, and rightly so. Cutting out of your diet foods that you've been eating for twenty, thirty or even sixty years can be both a thrilling and a scary process.

That being said, I don't want this chapter to instill food fear in you. I don't want you thinking that any prepackaged, store-bought or restaurant food is unhealthy, because that couldn't be further from the truth. In fact, in North America, we are pretty lucky when it comes to the availability of healthy options—although in smaller towns, the options for eating out are more limited. Still, it is always wisest to cook more of your own food.

I won't leave you fearing you have to ditch all these foods and then have nothing left to eat. The next chapter focuses on all the delicious foods you *can* eat, and the second half of my book is devoted to nourishing, detox-friendly and delicious recipes you can make yourself. You'll be pleased to know there is such an abundance of foods, especially those grown where you live, that are nutritious and yummy.

In this chapter I will guide you through the foods to ditch and teach you about food additives. It is important to know what to avoid because navigating the grocery store, and especially packaged foods, can be a confusing and frustrating experience. We simply cannot rely on our governments and big food companies to inform us what is healthy and what is not because far too many food additives are allowed on the market today that should not be in our food at all.

> This process of elimination really excites me because most people have no idea how good their body is meant to look and feel. Once you remove certain foods and food additives, you will likely get that glow and sparkle back that you may remember from your childhood or teenage years.

Most people just become satisfied with the status quo regarding how they feel—they feel "okay," so why should they change? If they don't get a cold or flu during the cooler months, they figure they are healthy. They assume that simply avoiding disease is the same as health. However, this couldn't be further from the truth. You should expect to thrive with great health and feel fantastic, not just "okay." And you can feel amazing when you nourish your body with the recipes in my book and take a break from the foods and additives described in this chapter. By removing these foods and additives, you give your body a chance to heal, reduce inflammation and realize how good it is truly designed to feel. It's not surprising that the word *heal* is part of the word *health*, is it?

If I had a penny for every client or Joyous 10-day detoxer who told me they never realized how good they could feel, and now that they've completed the detox they look better, they think better, they have lost weight, their skin is glowing, their pain has dramatically been reduced or completely vanished, I'd be a millionaire by now. The proof is in the (chia) pudding, my friends!

Taking a break from these foods or avoiding them permanently is guaranteed to yield great results. You don't need a double-blind placebo-controlled study to tell you that eating less crap and eating more whole foods will have dramatic and positive results.

Here are the top foods and food additives to ditch:

- refined sugar
- artificial sweeteners
- food additives
- dairy
- gluten
- peanuts
- unfermented soy
- corn
- alcohol
- coffee
- genetically modified organisms

To make things easier for you, none of the recipes in this book contains a single one of these ingredients. You won't even miss them, because you'll be so gosh darn satisfied!

REFINED SUGAR

I have great news for you: your life will become sweeter without sugar!

You may have heard me call sugar evil, and yes, it is evil. Sugar makes us crazy. It certainly made me feel like a crazy moody monster when I pounded back a small bag of chocolate-covered almonds every afternoon in my (pre-nutritionist) office job, but I was addicted. I know I'm not the only one. Every time I do an audience poll when I'm speaking and ask how many people feel addicted to and controlled by sugar, at least half the audience raises their hand. This doesn't surprise me, since sugar triggers the release of dopamine, a neurotransmitter that makes us feel good and is therefore very addictive.

Refined sugar is nutrient-dead. It contains no protein, vitamins, minerals, fibre or antioxidants. And I'm not talking only about the bagged white sugar you see in grocery stores, which is almost always derived from genetically modified sugar beets. Sugar is found in most packaged foods, from the obvious ones, such as pastries, cakes and candies, to the not so obvious sources, such as boxed cereals, granola and energy bars, as well as salad dressings and bottled sauces. It's a sneaky ingredient that comes in many different forms.

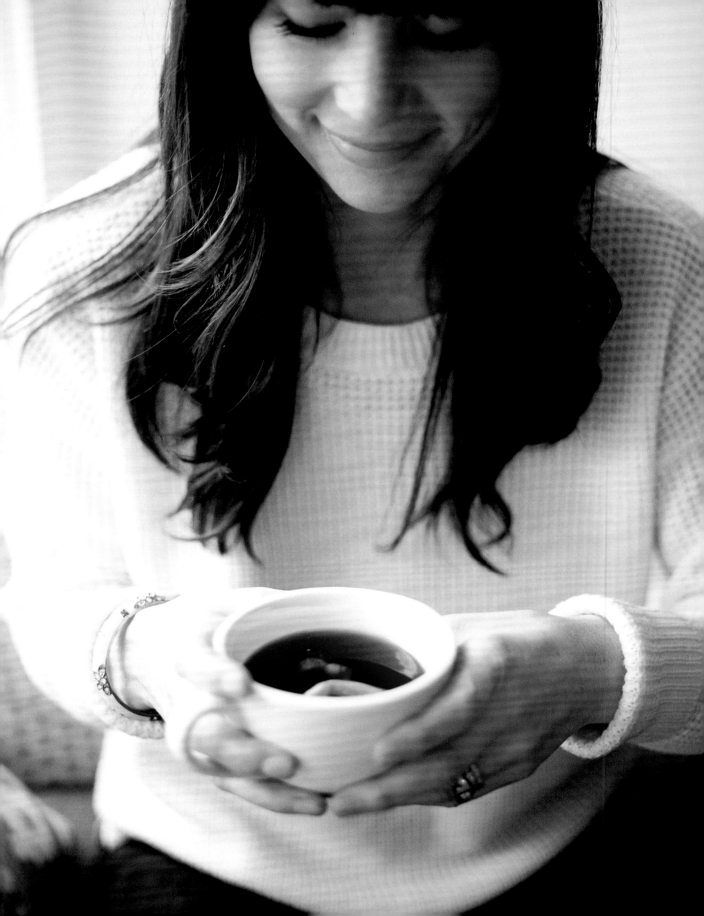

Sugar makes us fat

Researchers and healthcare practitioners all agree that sugar is making us sick and fat. It's not fat that makes us fat, as the experts used to tell us in the 1980s and '90s—it's sugar! When we eat too much sugar, the liver converts the excess to fat, and this extra fat is sent to the belly, hips and thighs for storage. It is not just the fattening of North America that sugar is largely responsible for. It's also linked to type 2 diabetes, insulin resistance, fatty liver disease, metabolic syndrome and all the diseases that are a result of these health problems, such as heart disease.

However, you are ultimately in control of what passes by your lips, so you can make informed decisions and simply avoid this food additive for the duration of the Joyous Detox.

What kinds of sugar am I talking about?

- **Monosaccharides, also known as "simple" or "refined" carbs or sugars**, are listed on food labels as **dextrose**, **fructose** and **glucose**. The primary difference between these is how your body metabolizes them. Fructose is a beast all on its own. In studies on rats and mice, if fructose hits the liver in a sufficient quantity (such as when you schlop agave all over your cereal), the liver will convert most of it to fat because it's *not* the preferred source of energy for the body. Agave can be up to 80 percent fructose. Eating foods high in fructose (especially high-fructose corn syrup) all the time can induce a condition known as insulin resistance and can lead to obesity and sugar cravings.

  Fructose found in fruit is different because it comes along with vitamins, minerals, enzymes, fibre and hundreds of phytonutrients that not only assist in assimilation but also have many other health benefits.

- **Disaccharides, also known as "complex sugars,"** are listed on a label as **sucrose**, **maltose** and **lactose**. Sucrose is the same thing as white table sugar (usually made from GMOs) and the most common ingredient that you'll find in traditional baking recipes. Sucrose is made from glucose and fructose.

  Brown sugar is no better. It is just sucrose with molasses added for colour.

You might be wondering if you can ever again eat something that contains sugars in it

While you are doing the Joyous Detox, I recommend that you avoid any sugar that ends in "-ose," except for fructose when it is naturally occurring in fruit. Additionally, some natural sweeteners, such as raw honey, contain fructose and other sugars. In moderation and in a "whole-food form," these sugars are fine. If you follow the recipes in the Joyous Detox, you will be able to avoid refined sugars with ease because you won't be eating any packaged foods. And you'll likely find your blood sugar is so balanced, you don't have any cravings for refined sugars.

Sugar alcohols—use in moderation

Sugar alcohols are one of many sugar substitutes that are especially popular in the health community today. Sugar alcohols are not actually sugar or alcohol but a hybrid of the two. Xylitol is probably the most popular, but there is also sorbitol, maltitol, mannitol and erythritol. Sugar alcohols come from plant sources but have to be chemically altered. They do not occur naturally.

Sugar alcohols are found in many "low-cal," "no sugar" and "diet" foods and drinks. This is because they are incompletely absorbed by your small intestine, so they provide fewer calories than sugar. But this also means that when used every day they can cause digestive problems, such as bloating, diarrhea and flatulence. You may notice that xylitol is used in many natural health products, such as toothpaste, mints and gum. In small quantities, and when you aren't swallowing large amounts, it's fine. In fact, xylitol in toothpaste can actually help prevent cavities, according to a study published in the *Journal of the California Dental Association* in 2003. I still wouldn't use these sugars as the main sugar substitute in baking, though. I recommend focusing on whole foods in their most natural state, which is why I haven't used any of these sugars in my recipes.

ARTIFICIAL SWEETENERS

You need to avoid all artificial sweeteners. Here's the low-down on these chemically derived, non-food substances.

Artificial sweeteners are big business in North America and may be especially attractive to those suffering from diabetes because artificial sweeteners do not affect blood sugar levels. (However, that's up for debate!) Because of our addiction to sweetness, several sugar substitutes are approved for use in Canada. The main ones include acesulfame potassium (or Ace-K), aspartame, cyclamate, saccharin and sucralose. The first thing I want you to know is that these are chemically manufactured molecules that do not exist in nature. There is nothing "food-ish or food-like" about them. And just like refined sugar, they contain absolutely no nutrients.

Ace-K

How to spot it: Read your labels because it's found in packaged baked goods, chewing gum, soft drinks and energy drinks.

Of all the artificial sweeteners available, Ace-K has received the least scrutiny— or perhaps it has just slipped through the cracks. It is derived from acetoacetic acid and fluorosulfonyl isocyanate, and it's two hundred times sweeter than table sugar. Ace-K is a potassium salt containing methylene chloride, a known carcinogen. There have been reports that Ace-K may contribute to hypoglycemia, which is ironic considering it's in many foods you may be choosing in order to avoid blood sugar imbalance issues in the first place.

Aspartame

How to spot it: Aspartame is branded as Equal and NutraSweet. It is often added to "zero-calorie" and "no-sugar" packaged foods such as desserts, yogurts and drinks.

Aspartame is a laboratory concoction of aspartic acid, phenylalanine and methanol. Aspartic acid accumulates in brain tissue, and researchers have been looking into the link with dysfunctions in the brain. The problem is that we don't really know what the cumulative effect of drinking diet pop or using aspartame in your coffee might be after thirty years of use. We do know that aspartame has resulted in an increase in brain tumours in animals, according to a study published in the *Journal of Neuropathology and Experimental Neurology*. Coincidentally, the increase in brain tumours in our society happened when aspartame was introduced in the 1970s.

It seems that the more we consume aspartame and the more we are exposed to its constituent chemicals, the higher our risk of experiencing negative side effects.

Even though the Canadian government considers aspartame safe—with cautions around usage for pregnant women—it is the subject of more health complaints than any other food additive.

Cyclamate

How to spot it: It is not allowed to be added to packaged foods and drinks, but you can find packets of it marketed as Sugar Twin, Sweet'N Low and Sucaryl.

Another man-made chemical! Cyclamate is the salt of a synthetic acid. (It was discovered in 1937 by a student at the University of Illinois while he was working in the lab on an anti-fever medication. He put his cigarette down on the lab bench, only to realize when he smoked it again that it tasted sweet from the chemical he had accidentally dipped it into.) Cyclamate is currently banned in the United States—but not in Canada—because it has a super-sketchy past. Some studies have linked it to bladder cancer, others have linked it to testicular atrophy in mice, and still others contradict these findings. But it remains a controversial food additive because so little is known about its long-term effects.

Saccharin

How to spot it: Packaged and sold as saccharin at grocery stores.

Saccharin is three hundred to four hundred times sweeter than sugar. It is available to purchase for baking but it is not allowed to be added to packaged foods or drinks in Canada. It is derived from coal tar, so you can bet there is nothing food-like about it. In the past it has been linked to cancer in rats, although this finding is controversial because scientists are not sure it can be duplicated in humans. Nevertheless, any food additive that "may" be linked to cancer should be avoided.

Sucralose

How to spot it: Splenda is the brand name of sucralose. It is often found alongside table sugar in restaurants and is also added to packaged foods and drinks.

Sucralose is six hundred times sweeter than sugar! Despite its deceptive name, it is not even remotely close to sugar. It is made by chlorinating sucrose, which completely changes its molecular structure. Initially, researchers said it worked as a zero-calorie sweetener because it was not absorbed in the digestive tract. Newer studies show that sucralose is in fact metabolized and can reduce good gut bacteria; when used in baking, it can release toxins called chloropropanols; and it can alter insulin and blood sugar levels. These findings were in studies done on rats, but keep in mind that the studies the U.S. Food and Drug Administration used to approve sucralose were also done on rats.

The bottom line on artificial sweeteners

When your brain detects a sweet taste on your tongue, it tells the body to expect nutrition. Researchers at the Center for Human Nutrition at Washington University School of Medicine in St. Louis found that simply detecting a sweet taste can elicit an insulin response in your body. When no nutrition is delivered—because artificial sweeteners are nutrient-dead man-made substances—your body doesn't feel satiated, and you will crave more food! This could be one of the main reasons that drinkers of diet pop actually tend to gain more fat, as shown in studies published in the *Journal of the American Geriatrics Society*.

> "I never thought I would be able to lose my addiction to sugar. The more I had, the more I wanted. To my surprise, after just cutting it out for ten days, I found I lost my appetite for it, and when I did reintroduce some sweet foods, I found them sickly sweet and just not enjoyable anymore." —Janet

So, no sugar and no artificial sweeteners. You're probably wondering what you *can* use to sweeten your food. More on that in chapter 4, when you learn to stock your kitchen joyously!

FOOD ADDITIVES

Now that you know about some of the most popular artificial sweeteners, which are food additives all on their own, let's talk about some other additives to watch out for. You've probably seen carrageenan, xanthan gum and food colouring listed on food labels. These are examples of popular food additives. And then there's transglutaminase, also known as "meat glue," and the dyes given to salmon to make their colour more appealing. Some of these additives are harmless, but many others are suspicious and some can cause a variety of health problems.

The problem with food additives (a.k.a. chemical substances) is that no one has ever studied the effect of ingesting a cocktail of substances in combination with each other. We simply don't know what effect they might have after years of ingesting the sheer volume of packaged foods that is our food system today.

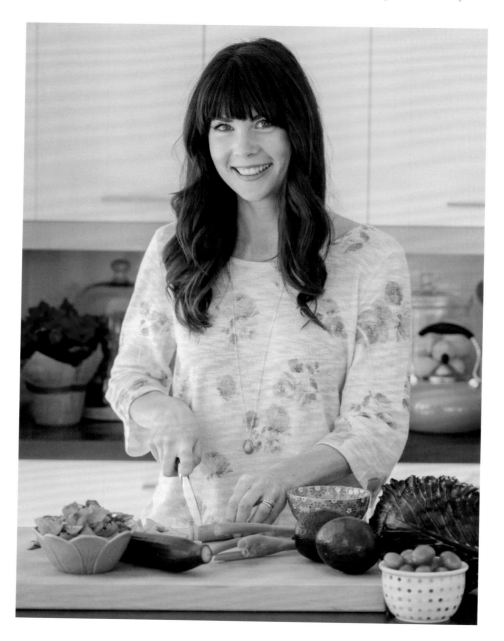

According to Health Canada, "a food additive is any chemical substance that is added to food during preparation or storage and either becomes a part of the food or affects its characteristics for the purpose of achieving a particular technical effect." In Canada, more than 850 food additives are registered for use, and the list is growing. Food additives are used as anti-caking agents, food colourings, emulsifiers, gelling and thickening agents, preservatives, you name it. According to the Center for Science in the Public Interest, in North America more than ten thousand different chemicals—both natural and artificial—are added to our food. This goes beyond approved food additives and includes chemicals such as those on the FDA's Generally Recognized as Safe (GRAS) list, natural and artificial flavourings, pesticides and indirect chemicals from packaging and the environment.

The government classifies some additives as GRAS because they are assumed safe in food and not required to be reviewed and properly approved. It's up to manufacturers to decide whether these compounds are safe by relying on expert panels, without any input from the FDA. This results in huge loopholes in the system for potentially harmful additives to slip through the cracks. Scary and frustrating, isn't it?

One challenge with food additives is that the sheer number of them makes it difficult to determine what specific chemical could be harming you. Chances are, if you eat packaged and processed foods regularly, you may be affected by multiple additives, making it harder to determine specific triggers of symptoms. Many people have reported digestive problems from carrageenan, allergic reactions to food dyes (especially hyperactivity in children), neurological symptoms from flavour enhancers, headaches from artificial sweeteners—the list goes on.

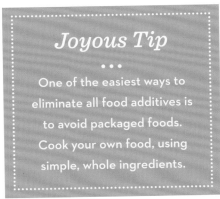

Joyous Tip

• • •

One of the easiest ways to eliminate all food additives is to avoid packaged foods. Cook your own food, using simple, whole ingredients.

During your detox, you may find your symptoms completely disappear because your body is not coming into contact with any food additives to act as triggers. On page 12 are the Dirty Dozen food additives according to the Environmental Working Group. Unfortunately, the foods noted as on the GRAS list are not always listed on food labels.

DIRTY DOZEN FOOD ADDITIVES

FOOD ADDITIVE	HEALTH CONCERN	HOW TO SPOT IT
Nitrites and nitrates—preservative, colouring agent and flavour enhancer	Nitrites, which can form from nitrates, react with naturally occurring components of proteins called amines. This reaction can form nitrosamines, which are known cancer-causing compounds.	Cured meats: bacon, salami, hot dogs, sausages
Potassium bromate—used to strengthen bread and cracker dough and help it rise during baking	Causes tumours in animals, is toxic to the kidneys and can cause DNA damage.	Store-bought baked goods
Propylene paraben—food preservative; GRAS	An endocrine-disrupting chemical. Acts as a weak synthetic estrogen and can alter the expression of genes, including those in breast cancer cells.	Store-bought tortillas, muffins; in food dyes; in packaging used for dairy, meat and vegetables
Butylated hydroxyanisole (BHA)—preservative; GRAS	Hormone disrupter and possible human carcinogen.	Chips and preserved meat, as well as many other foods that contain fats
Butylated hydroxytoluene (BHT)—preservative and cousin to BHA; GRAS	Linked to developmental effects, thyroid changes, lung and liver tumours, and cancer in animals.	Often added to foods that also contain BHA
Propyl gallate—preservative; GRAS	Possible endocrine disrupter; associated with brain tumour formation in animals.	Sausages and lard
Theobromine—alkaloid found in chocolate that has effects similar to caffeine	May cause reproductive and developmental effects.	Bread, cereal, sports drinks, cocoa products and snacks
Flavour ingredients—used to enhance the flavour of foods	Any time you see "natural" or "artificial" flavour listed on a label, beware. This can mean a whole host of different ingredients that food manufacturers do not have to disclose. It also means you have no idea if the food contains a chemical you are sensitive to. Unless the label says "certified organic natural flavours," you can't be certain there are no genetically modified or synthetic ingredients.	Packaged foods
Artificial colours—used to increase the visual appeal of foods that have little nutritional value	Various colouring agents have been linked to hyperactivity in children and to tumours, and may even cause cancer.	Highly processed foods like chips and candy tend to contain artificial colours. Read the labels of any packaged food.
Diacetyl—flavouring agent	Associated with a severe and irreversible respiratory condition.	Microwave popcorn, dairy products, products with butterscotch and maple flavouring and fruit flavourings such as strawberry and raspberry
Phosphates—used to leaven baked goods, reduce acid and improve moisture retention and tenderness in processed meats	High phosphorus in the body is linked to heart disease.	Found in more than 20,000 food products (check the EWG Food Score Database)
Aluminum additives—stabilizers in processed foods	Associated with neurological effects including Alzheimer's.	Additives containing aluminum, such as sodium aluminum phosphate and sodium aluminum sulphate, are used as stabilizers in many processed foods.

Source: Environmental Working Group

DAIRY

The "milk does a body good" marketing campaign from the '90s and early 2000s did a fantastic job of convincing millions of people that milk is the only health food they'd ever need. This is extremely misleading. Our government would even have us believe that milk is essential for our health and vitality; it's given a prominent place in our food guide and promoted as the best source of calcium for strong bones. But thousands of people who have taken a break from milk and milk products, or eliminated them completely, have experienced many benefits, from clearer skin to improved digestion and even weight loss.

Dairy products—including milk, yogurt and cheese—are best avoided during the Joyous Detox because they contain casein and whey protein. Both these proteins are very common allergens and provoke food sensitivities.

Despite there being no evidence supporting the claim that dairy is mucus-forming, simply ask anyone with sinus problems or excessive mucus if cutting out dairy made a difference. I've had hundreds of clients benefit from cutting out cow's milk. Additionally, some forms of dairy may increase levels of inflammatory chemicals in the body. Inflammation leads to a whole array of health issues, including blood sugar imbalance, insulin resistance and type 2 diabetes. Dairy is definitely something you want to avoid while detoxing.

Many dairy products, especially cow's milk products, are highly processed through both pasteurization and homogenization, leaving them sterile and hard to digest. Many yogurt products contain little or no good bacteria after being pasteurized and contain added sugar and artificial ingredients. When you are not on the detox, goat's and sheep's milk products are great alternatives to cow's milk products because they have much less casein protein and are therefore lower on the allergenic scale.

Cow's dairy, particularly liquid cow's milk, is also linked to skin problems ranging from eczema to acne, as shown in research conducted by the Department of Nutrition, Harvard School of Public Health. Any inflammatory response triggered by food may appear as a reaction on the skin. Many people see huge improvements in their skin and digestion after just a few days off dairy.

What about butter? You may use pure ghee on this detox, which is clarified butter, meaning all the protein has been removed and you are left with the pure fat. Be sure to purchase certified organic ghee. When you are not detoxing, butter in moderation is fine. In fact, it can be quite helpful for building a strong immune system because it contains fatty acids. Butter generally doesn't cause the same reactions in people as other cow's dairy products.

If you're concerned about your calcium intake, see the Frequently Asked Questions on page 93 for a list of dairy-free foods that contain calcium.

GLUTEN

Gluten-free foods have become extremely popular over the past few years. This is because many people benefit from taking a break from cereals, pasta, bread and the like. Gluten is the protein found in wheat, rye and barley. It is another common food allergen/sensitivity, just like dairy, and it is best avoided while detoxing. Even if you do not have celiac disease, you can still have gluten intolerance.

According to Beyond Celiac (formerly the National Foundation for Celiac Awareness), about 18 million Americans have non-celiac gluten sensitivity. These are people who tested negative for celiac disease but found their symptoms lessened or disappeared altogether after they removed gluten from their diet.

Gluten has been linked to insulin resistance. Eating just two pieces of whole wheat toast can spike insulin levels to those equivalent to eating 2 tbsp (30 mL) of sugar, according to Dr. William Davis, author of *Wheat Belly*. There are so many delicious recipes on the detox, you won't even miss wheat bread or white-flour pastries!

When you consider the Standard American Diet, it's not surprising that two of the most common food sensitivities are gluten and dairy. Most people's diets are full of bread and cheese. Eating the same foods day after day and year after year can cause you to become sensitive or intolerant to them. (The same is true of

> ### *Joyous Tip*
> • • •
> Not all foods labelled "gluten-free" are healthier than their gluten-containing counterparts. In fact, there is a whole raft of gluten-free junk foods that are best avoided. As always, read your labels and avoid foods containing refined sugars and food additives, gluten-free or not.

healthy foods, such as apples and leafy greens, but those contain fewer allergenic proteins than dairy and gluten.)

PEANUTS

Peanuts are a very common allergen. Even if you are not allergic to them, you can still be sensitive to them. They are high in a mould called aflatoxin and are best avoided, especially if you have a compromised immune system or an autoimmune disease.

UNFERMENTED SOY

Unfermented soy is a common allergen that is added to thousands of packaged foods. When soy became popular about fifteen years ago, many touted it as the new best health food because of its high protein content, making it ideal for vegetarians and vegans. Unfortunately, this misconception that it was the perfect food meant that food manufacturers started adding it to everything, from cereal to chocolate. Manufacturers love it because it's a cheap filler that boosts protein content. However, the resulting overconsumption of unfermented soy has led to soy allergies and sensitivities.

Unfermented soy is problematic because it contains many anti-nutrients. Among these are phytates, which reduce the absorption of minerals; enzyme inhibitors, which prevent digestive enzymes from breaking down carbohydrates and proteins; and goitrogens, which may suppress thyroid function. People most at risk of negative effects from unfermented soy include infants being fed soy formula, vegetarians eating a high-soy diet, those with hypothyroidism and women in menopause.

When soy is properly fermented, its phytates, enzyme inhibitors and goitrogens are neutralized, making it a food that is easily digested and health-promoting. So whether or not you're detoxing, the best form of soy to eat is fermented, including tempeh, miso, tamari and natto. Always make sure the soy you eat is certified organic, because more than 90 percent of soy crops are genetically modified and heavily sprayed with pesticides.

CORN

Corn is similar to soy in that it is added to most packaged foods as a cheap filler. If this is a new concept to you, I highly recommend the movie *King Corn*! Just like soy, corn is commonly genetically modified. It spikes blood sugar and can be inflammatory. I suggest you avoid all foods containing corn for the duration of the Joyous Detox. Beyond detoxing, always be sure to buy certified organic corn.

ALCOHOL

The body treats alcohol as a toxin, and it is processed by the liver as a waste product that must be eliminated. Of course, wine does have some benefits, such as antioxidants, but for the duration of the Joyous Detox, I recommend you avoid all forms of alcohol.

COFFEE

Caffeine, the stimulating component in coffee that North Americans are addicted to, is considered a drug and a food additive by the U.S. Food and Drug Administration. Your body craves it because it has mood-boosting properties.

When detoxing, the goal is to give your liver a break from having to process chemicals. Caffeine is detoxed by the liver, which draws on various nutrients to do this effectively. You may notice that matcha green tea is in a few of my recipes, but it contains a variety of other nutrients that support the body and provide a "clean energy."

If you are a coffee drinker and you're wondering how to effectively cut it out during the Joyous Detox, see page 96 for guidance on how to do a coffee detox and avoid the negative effects of quitting cold turkey.

GENETICALLY MODIFIED ORGANISMS (GMOS)

Introduced in the 1990s, genetically modified (or genetically engineered) ingredients can now be found in more than three-quarters of processed foods in North American supermarkets, according to the Center for Food Safety. Genetic modification of a food is the direct manipulation of the organism's genome using biotechnology—in other words, inserting, deleting or mutating the gene of the organism, often using genes from another species. There is nothing "natural" about this.

Polls show that 93 percent of Americans want the right to know if there are GMOs in their food. More than sixty countries now have mandatory labelling, but here in Canada and the United States, consumers are left in the dark. Food manufacturers are concerned that if they are required to label GMOs, people won't buy their products. But I think consumers deserve the choice.

These are just some of the problems with genetically modified foods:

- **Major increase in the use of chemical herbicides.** Genetically engineered crops are designed to withstand heavy doses of synthetic chemicals such as glyphosate. Glyphosate use increased 527 million pounds between 1996 and 2012. This chemical can now be found in our air, food and water. It may cause many health problems in both children and adults. It has been linked to brain tumours, birth defects and ADHD in children.

- **Increase in superweeds.** There are now seven different glyphosate-resistant superweeds. Nature is smart. If you create a synthetic chemical to kill pests and weeds, these organisms will eventually outwit you and come back stronger.

- **More toxic herbicides.** To control the growth of superweeds, farmers now have to resort to using more toxic herbicides. Many of these herbicides are linked to cancer, Parkinson's disease and reproductive problems, according to research by the Environmental Working Group.

- **Few safety studies.** The Canadian government requires strict safety studies before drugs reach the market, and there are also strict regulations on health food supplements, but there are no mandated safety studies for GMOs. This means that GMO crops have not been tested for whether they can cause cancer, for harm to fetuses or for risks over the long term to animals or humans.

- **Cross-contamination.** As the acres of GMO farm fields increase at an astronomical rate, organic farmers struggle to prevent cross-contamination of their crops by genetically modified seeds or pollen spread by wind, insects, floods and machinery. Genetically modified contamination has become a major issue for organic growers and has resulted in a major loss of profit by organic farmers.

These are the four most common genetically modified
ingredients in packaged foods:

1. **Field corn and corn-derived ingredients.** Most of this crop is grown
    for animal feed, but approximately 12 percent is processed to corn flour,
    high-fructose corn syrup, cornstarch, masa, cornmeal and corn oil that
    end up in foods.
2. **Soybeans and soy-derived ingredients.** All food products that
    contain soy proteins, soybean oil, soy milk, soy flour, soy sauce, tofu
    or soy lecithin have been made with genetically modified ingredients,
    unless they are certified organic or labelled "GMO-free."
3. **Sugar.** More than half of all sugar produced in the United States comes
    from sugar beets, of which 95 percent are GMO.
4. **Vegetable oils.** Nearly all vegetable oils, including canola oil, cottonseed
    oil, soybean oil and corn oil, are genetically modified, unless certified
    organic or labelled "GMO-free."

These are the three most commonly
genetically modified foods:

1. Hawaiian papaya
2. zucchini and yellow summer squash (from the U.S.)
3. sweet corn

The only way to avoid GMOs is to purchase certified organic foods or foods
labelled with the "NON-GMO PROJECT VERIFIED" seal. Look for these seals
on package labels. On produce, simply look for the number 9 at the start of
the PLU code, as this indicates organic, and GMOs are strictly prohibited in
organic farming.

It's possible that by the time you are reading this there will be even more genetically modified foods on supermarket shelves, including salmon, apples, flaxseeds, plums, potatoes, radicchio, rice, tomatoes and wheat.

Okay, so I've suggested you avoid quite a number of foods and food additives, but remember that you have a plethora of delicious and nourishing recipes in chapter 6 that are completely free of these foods and food additives. You'll be so well nourished, you won't even miss these foods.

Joyous Affirmation

I realize that wellness is a journey and as each new day dawns I welcome new and positive health habits and let go of those that do not serve me well.

2

JOYOUS DETOX
SUPERFOODS

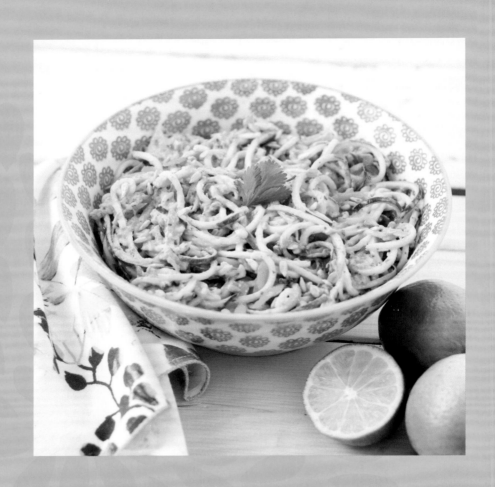

Aside from the recipes in chapter 6, this is one of the most important chapters in *Joyous Detox* because, as I mentioned earlier, most detoxes and cleanses focus far too much on what to avoid, and I'm not a fan of that approach. I would rather you focus on all the foods you *can* eat, because when you fill up on healthy, detox-friendly foods, you'll have less room in your belly for the bad stuff! When you nourish your body with nutrient-dense food, you can banish cravings for good.

These are my favourite Joyous Detox superfoods, which you'll learn about in this chapter:

- almonds
- apples
- avocados
- beetroots
- dark berries
- chia
- cinnamon
- cruciferous vegetables
- fennel
- fermented foods
- garlic
- ginger
- grapefruit
- hemp seeds
- herbs
- legumes
- lemons (and limes)
- matcha green tea
- oats
- onions
- quinoa
- sea vegetables
- sunflower seeds
- turmeric

In this chapter, I'm going to introduce you to some "detox superfoods." Just because these foods are considered detox superfoods doesn't mean they are recommended only while you are detoxing. Also, just because they are considered superfoods doesn't necessarily mean that they are exotic or expensive, or they should be eaten only while you are following a detox. In fact, you can grow some of these foods in your backyard, and I recommend you eat them every day!

The reason I suggest you eat these foods every day is because your body is constantly trying to rid itself of chemicals and toxins, whether they are endogenous (created by your body itself, as a by-product of cellular metabolism) or exogenous (taken in through outside sources). Eating detox superfoods daily will support all your detox systems, especially the master organ of detoxification, your liver. An awesome side benefit of eating these foods daily is that they'll help your skin glow and your inner beauty shine, thanks to a clean and healthy digestive system!

> ## Joyous Tip
>
> • • •
>
> Before you dive into learning about these superfoods, please note that every fruit and vegetable contains vitamins, minerals, antioxidants and thousands of phytonutrients that support your health and vitality. Just because something is not listed here doesn't mean that it's not a superfood. I don't want you to assume that the foods I've listed below are the only foods you should be eating. For instance, I don't list carrots as a detox superfood, but I've included them in a variety of recipes because they are an inexpensive vegetable with a plethora of health benefits.

The health benefits of these detox superfoods are extensive. I am mainly going to touch on the benefits that relate to detoxification. Of course, there are far more health benefits to eating these superfoods than what I've listed here.

With each detox superfood, I've suggested corresponding recipes for you to try so that detoxing is as delicious as possible. In fact, I'm pretty confident you won't even feel like you're detoxing, because everything is going to taste so darn yummy.

ALMONDS

Raw or roasted, whole, or as a butter or milk, almonds are a nutrient-dense addition to any salad or smoothie and they are a portable healthy snack you can take anywhere. When you roast almonds, you do limit some of their healthy fat content. But let's face it, eating almonds, raw or roasted, instead of reaching for a bag of chips is a step in the right direction.

Joyous Detox facts about almonds

- **High in fibre.** Almonds help you feel fuller longer and are essential for healthy elimination.
- **Great source of protein.** Almonds contain 6 g of protein per ounce. In fact, a handful of almonds has as much protein as one egg! This easily digested protein helps stabilize blood sugar and prevent future sugar cravings.
- **Great source of vitamin E.** Vitamin E is a fat-soluble antioxidant that neutralizes free radicals and is a potent anti-inflammatory nutrient.
- **Wonderful source of bone-building nutrients.** Almonds contain calcium and magnesium, which are essential for healthy, strong bones and teeth.
- **Healthy fats.** Almonds are a great source of anti-inflammatory monounsaturated fatty acids.

I use a variety of nuts and seeds in my recipes. Variety is the key. I've highlighted almonds here because they are such a versatile nut to use in cooking, but there are many other tasty, nutrient-dense nuts and seeds.

How to enjoy them: Almonds come in many forms—whole, ground and milk—which makes them a versatile ingredient in recipes. The Baked Brown Rice Pudding on page 250 is made with almond milk instead of dairy milk, making it ideal for the Joyous Detox. Any smoothie can be made with almond milk, as it adds a creamy texture without any belly bloat. Be sure to try making your own almond milk; see Nutty Milk on page 148.

APPLES

My favourite fruit—aside from avocados, of course! I always recommend choosing certified organic apples when possible because apples are on the "Dirty Dozen" list. This list identifies fruits and vegetables that have the highest levels of pesticide residues compared with other produce. If you get the chance, go apple picking in the fall and you'll get the freshest and most nutrient-dense apples possible.

Joyous Detox facts about apples

- **Rich in insoluble fibre.** This type of fibre helps to cleanse and detoxify the digestive system and provide food for good gut bacteria.

- **Rich in a soluble fibre called pectin.** Pectin supports peristalsis (the muscle movement that pushes waste through the digestive system) and therefore the excretion of toxic waste, as well as providing food for good gut bacteria to thrive on.
- **Hormonally balancing.** A source of D-glucaric acid, which helps the body eliminate estrogen-like chemicals and potential carcinogens, including heavy metals.
- **High in vitamin C.** This is an essential nutrient for effective detoxification because it protects the liver from free radicals that could otherwise cause damage.
- **Blood sugar balancing and low in the glycemic index.** Apples combined with almond butter make a great snack to banish cravings.
- **Super hydrating.** Apples increase the moisture level of your skin.

How to enjoy them: The Apple Pie Bites on page 260 are a super snack to enjoy while detoxing because you won't actually feel like you're, well, detoxing. I also love Ma McCarthy's Baked Apples and Pears with Coconut Butter on page 249. Because apples are hydrating, they are ideal for smoothies and juices, so try the Rejuvenate Me Smoothie on page 146 and the Green Sparkle Smoothie on page 139.

AVOCADOS

You'll find many avocado-based recipes on my blog and in this book because who doesn't love the buttery creaminess of an avocado? Unless you are allergic or sensitive to it, avocado is a detox superfood, so stock up your kitchen every week. Avocados work wonders for making smoothies and sauces extra creamy, and they're a great substitute for dairy, as you will see in the recipes chapter.

Joyous Detox facts about avocados

- **Good fats.** Avocados contain a good kind of fat called monounsaturated fats—particularly oleic acid, which is beneficial for its anti-inflammatory action. Good fat keeps your cells well lubricated and your skin moisturized. It also helps keep you satiated after a meal.
- **Good source of fibre.** There are 10 g of fibre in a 1-cup (250 mL) serving. Fibre slows the release of glucose into the bloodstream.

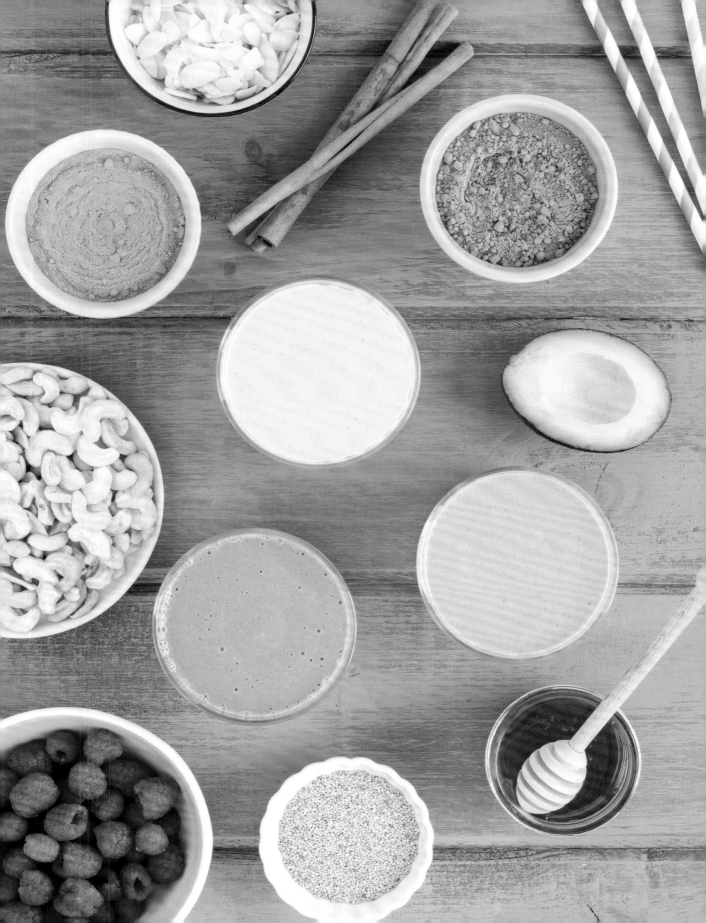

- Nutrient-dense. A good source of vitamin C, which protects your body from the free radical damage that toxic waste products can cause. Great source of all the B vitamins (except B_{12}). B vitamins are essential for many of the detoxification processes that happen in the liver. And finally, a good source of vitamin E, an antioxidant vitamin that works synergistically with vitamin C (among others).

How to enjoy them: It might surprise you that avocados are equally delicious at breakfast, such as in the Blueberry Bliss Smoothie Bowl on page 147, and at lunch or dinner—try the Mint Guacamole Lettuce Wraps on page 220. If you love devilled eggs, try the Guacamole Devilled Eggs on page 120. When zucchini are in season, I love making Zucchini Noodles with Avocado Cream Sauce on page 239.

BEETROOTS

Beets have been known for hundreds of years as a purifier and a blood builder. They are one of the first foods many people think of when they consider adding detox-friendly foods to their diet. Beets are a fantastic way to check your "transit time" to ensure the timely elimination of waste products from your body. You might have read about that in my first book, *Joyous Health*. If not, see the Frequently Asked Questions on page 93 to learn more about checking your transit time.

And don't toss out the beet greens on top! They are a rich source of vitamin C and considered a bitter food. Bitter foods—such as leafy greens—stimulate the flow of bile, which aids in detoxification. Beet juice is also cleansing and extremely anti-inflammatory.

Joyous Detox facts about beets

- Liver lover. Beets are a rich source of betaine, which is an essential compound for proper liver function and protection from harmful toxins. Betaine improves liver function by thinning the bile, allowing it to flow freely through the liver and into the small intestine, carrying toxins and waste products with it.

- Incredible detox food. Beets are rich in a group of phytonutrients called betalains that give beets their rich colour and also support phase two liver detoxification.
- Rich in antioxidants and anti-inflammatory compounds.
- Great source of fibre. Fibre encourages the elimination of waste products.

How to enjoy them: Since beets are one of nature's best liver cleansers and protectors, I recommend eating them at least once a week, raw or cooked. My favourite way to eat them raw is to just grate them into a salad. Try the Give Thanks Mason Jar Salad on page 190 or the Everything but the Kitchen Sink Salad with Creamy Dijon Dressing on page 192. Combined with strawberries in a juice they are absolutely delicious; try the Beet and Strawberry Detox Juice on page 151.

DARK BERRIES

Dark berries, including blueberries, blackberries, cherries, raspberries and strawberries, are delicious. There's a reason they're called nature's candy! When fresh berries are in season, I eat them nearly every day. I will often buy them in bulk from the farmers' market and freeze extras so I can enjoy them all year long. Berries are one of my favourite fruits to add to smoothies and sprinkle on top of granola because they provide such a megawatt dose of nutrients.

Joyous Detox facts about dark berries
- Liver lover. Dark berries are high in antioxidant bioflavonoids (such as anthocyanins and ellagic acid) and dietary fibre, all of which have liver-protecting and detoxifying properties.
- Nutrient-dense. Very high in vitamin A, vitamin C, folate and choline.
- Prevent sugar cravings. Relatively low on the glycemic index, dark berries are an ideal snack food because they won't spike your blood sugar levels and promote cravings for sugar.

How to enjoy them: I'm a total pancake monster, which is why the Buckwheat Pancakes with Warmed Blueberries on page 105 are my go-to—and yes, they are detox friendly! Blueberry Chia Jam on page 178 is truly an everyday detox superfood that can be slathered on and enjoyed with just about anything, from gluten-free toast to the Coconut Yogurt Parfait with Chia Jam on page 110.

CHIA

Chia is a tiny seed first used by the Aztecs in 3500 BC. It was even used as currency in ancient times because it is such a valuable food source. Chia absorbs liquid easily, so it is best known for its ability to thicken puddings, jams and smoothies. Don't let its size fool you into thinking it's not a nutrition powerhouse, because it is!

Joyous Detox facts about chia

- No belly bloat. Chia is higher in fibre than wheat bran and will not cause bloating, which many bran cereals do. In fact 3 tbsp (45 mL) of chia contains 11 g of fibre, and it's almost all soluble fibre, which is why chia absorbs liquid so well. Soluble fibre is excellent for digestion and detox because it absorbs toxins in the digestive tract. Bonus: it is known to help lower cholesterol and triglyceride levels.
- Keeps you feeling full. Although chia is not a "miracle" weight-loss food, the fibre in it helps to promote feelings of satiety, preventing overeating.
- Totally gluten-free.
- Anti-inflammatory. Rich source of a plant-based omega-3 fatty acid called alpha-linolenic acid, which is anti-inflammatory.

How to enjoy it: I include chia seeds in many recipes in this book because they are such an incredible detox superfood. My favourite recipes include the chia seed drinks on pages 133–134 as a great way to hydrate when you're on the go or to tide you over until your next meal, and the chia jams on pages 178–179 as a quick snack. But my favourite chia seed recipe is definitely the Raspberry Vanilla Bean Chia Pudding on page 259!

CINNAMON

Many of my dessert and smoothie recipes include cinnamon because it adds a natural sweetness without adding sugar or calories. When cutting sugar out of your diet, it helps to include spices such as cinnamon so that you still get the sweet taste but without all the negative effects of sugar.

Joyous Detox facts about cinnamon

- **Antibacterial and antifungal.** Cinnamon has been studied for its ability to help stop the growth of bacteria and fungi, including the commonly problematic yeast *Candida albicans*. Candida can be dreadful when you're trying to control cravings because it increases the need for sugar, since the yeast feeds on sugar.
- **Slows digestion.** Slows the rate at which the stomach empties after meals, reducing the rise in blood sugar after eating.
- **Aids elimination.** An excellent source of fibre and a good source of calcium. Both calcium and fibre can bind to bile salts, which contain toxic waste, and help remove them from the body.

How to enjoy it: Cinnamon can be sprinkled on top of just about anything, from smoothies to juices, or incorporated into recipes such as the Apple Pie Bites on page 260 or the Best Ever Cinnamon Flaxseed Bread on page 127.

CRUCIFEROUS VEGETABLES: ARUGULA, BRUSSELS SPROUTS, CABBAGE (GREEN AND RED), KALE, BROCCOLI, CAULIFLOWER, RUTABAGA AND TURNIPS

I cannot say enough about the healthiness of this group of vegetables, especially when it comes to detoxification. Unfortunately, these veggies have a bad reputation because most adults recall being forced to eat them as children and can still remember their rotten, sulphurous smell from being overcooked. These foods should not be overlooked (or overcooked!). They have a potent dose of nutrients that makes them detox superstars, and they are cancer-preventative foods. I suggest mixing up your diet and eating both raw and cooked cruciferous vegetables.

Joyous Detox facts about cruciferous vegetables

- **Cancer fighters.** Cruciferous vegetables have a proven track record in lowering the risk of certain cancers. They contain glucosinolates, a group of phytonutrients whose main job is to detoxify harmful compounds that could otherwise damage DNA and cause cancer.

- Toxin fighters. Two compounds made from glucosinolates, sulforaphane and indole-3-carbinol, promote the release of various toxin-fighting enzymes and neutralize potential cancer-causing substances.
- High concentrations of vitamin C, an essential nutrient for detoxification.
- Protect the liver. A rich source of beta-carotene, the precursor to vitamin A that helps to protect the liver against disease and harmful toxins. Cruciferous vegetables also contain many phytonutrient antioxidants, including quercetin, caffeic acid and ferulic acid, which help to protect cells and reduce inflammation.
- Anti-inflammatory. They contain not only anti-inflammatory glucosinolates but are also high in omega-3 fatty acids, in particular alpha-linolenic acid, a building block of inflammation-reducing EPA, an essential fatty acid.

How to enjoy them: I love the crunch of Purple and Green Cabbage Slaw on page 204 and the flavours in the Superfood Salad with Creamy Dressing on page 201. For cold winter nights, Cheesy Cauliflower Casserole on page 214 is the perfect comfort food yet still detoxifying.

FENNEL

My first introduction to fennel was as a tea. Even though I loved the taste of black licorice as a kid, I hated fennel until I started eating it raw or in forms other than tea. My husband, Walker, used to work with a lot of Italian guys and they would bring it to the office and eat it raw like celery! Once I learned how to cook with fennel, I fell in love with it. Then I learned about all the detoxifying benefits of this amazing superfood.

Joyous Detox facts about fennel

- Rich in antioxidants and anti-inflammatory compounds. Fennel contains the flavonoids rutin and quercetin, as well as various kaempferol glycosides, all of which give it strong antioxidant activity. Contains an anti-inflammatory phytonutrient called anethole.

- Rich in vitamin C. An excellent source of vitamin C, the body's primary water-soluble antioxidant, which is known for its ability to detoxify bacterial toxins, drugs, environmental toxins and heavy metals. High levels of vitamin C also help the detoxification process by rebalancing intestinal flora and strengthening the immune system.
- Great for elimination. A very good source of fibre, which increases elimination of toxins from the body, and also adds bulk to your stool, helping waste move faster through your gut.

How to enjoy it: Citrus Fennel Salad with Toasted Sunflower Seeds on page 184 is always a crowd-pleaser because it's super flavourful and refreshing. One of my favourite mains is Walker's Chicken with Fennel, Orange and Mint on page 240.

FERMENTED FOODS

From sauerkraut to kimchi, from kombucha to apple cider vinegar, the variety of fermented foods is as extensive as their health benefits. Fermented foods are extremely easy for your body to digest and absolutely delicious! Whenever you buy fermented or pickled vegetables, make sure the label does not list vinegar as an ingredient. If it does, it has not been properly fermented using traditional methods.

Joyous Detox facts about fermented foods

- Digestion friendly. Fermented foods improve gut health, which reduces bloating and constipation.
- Aid good bacteria. They help feed good bacteria and encourage them to flourish. Good bacteria help to break down toxins and waste products in the digestive system, which enhances detoxification.
- Ease digestion. When a food is fermented, the anti-nutrients (such as phytic acid, enzyme inhibitors and lectins) are removed, allowing for easier digestion.
- Aid nutrient absorption. They increase the bioavailability of nourishing vitamins, minerals, amino acids and carbohydrates.

How to enjoy them: You may be new to fermented foods, but they have been eaten in many cultures for hundreds of years. Spring-Inspired Kimchi on page 207 is best enjoyed as a condiment; I love it with scrambled eggs. Sauerkraut is another nourishing fermented food, and it's surprisingly easy to make your Crunch-tastic Sauerkraut on page 205.

GARLIC

Garlic not only adds a wonderful flavour to dishes but is bursting with health benefits, and not just those that enhance detoxification but also antibacterial ones. Garlic is known for its many heart-health benefits.

Joyous Detox facts about garlic

- Nutrient-dense. Garlic is an excellent source of a variety of vitamins and minerals, including vitamins B_1, B_6 and C, copper, manganese, selenium, phosphorus and calcium.
- Natural antibiotic. Aids the body in eliminating bacteria and viruses thanks to the sulphur compounds that give garlic its aroma. In fact, researchers at Washington State University found that a garlic compound called diallyl sulphide was more effective than antibiotics at killing *Campylobacter* bacteria, a common cause of food poisoning.
- Liver lover. Contains sulphur compounds that support detoxification pathways and protect the liver.
- Detox for the lungs. Cleanses the respiratory tract by expelling mucus buildup in the lungs and sinuses.

How to enjoy it: No pesto would be complete without garlic; try the Chicken Pesto Frittata on page 107 or the Almond Arugula Lemon Pesto on page 196 and get a healthy dose of garlic.

GINGER

Ginger adds a spicy kick to any dish, sweet or savoury. It is an absolute detox superfood kitchen staple because it is so incredibly versatile. In the cooler months, I love adding chunks of fresh ginger to hot water with lemon or using it in a fresh juice. Not only does it have detox benefits but it's effective at boosting your immune system too.

Joyous Detox facts about ginger

- Increases heat in the body. Ginger promotes healthy sweating, which can aid in detoxification.
- Reduces gas and bloating. An excellent carminative (a substance that promotes the elimination of intestinal gas) and intestinal spasmolytic (a substance that relaxes and soothes the intestinal tract).
- Anti-inflammatory. Contains very potent anti-inflammatory compounds called gingerols.

How to enjoy it: Raw ginger can be added to any smoothie or juice for some zippy zing! My personal favourite is Detox Ginger Tea on page 131 because it is a fantastic way to detox and relax. The Sesame Orange Quinoa Bowl on page 230 is my go-to when entertaining because it's always a hit.

GRAPEFRUIT

Even grapefruit's scientific name, *Citrus × paradisi*, evokes sunshine and images of a tropical paradise, just like its flavour! Grapefruit packs all the same nutritional punch as its citrusy cousins lemons and limes (we'll meet them in a bit), but certain grapefruit varieties also have added nutritional and detoxification benefits, so choose carefully when you're at the grocery store.

Joyous Detox facts about grapefruit

- Rich in antioxidants. Grapefruit are especially high in that all-important antioxidant, vitamin C, and in carotenoids like lycopene, which help fight cell damage induced by free radicals.
- Aid detox. Contain the detoxifying phytonutrients limonoids, which can inhibit tumour formation.
- Digestion friendly. A source of the detoxifying soluble fibre pectin, which helps keep things moving through your digestive tract.

How to enjoy them: Grapefruit can be substituted for lemons in many recipes, especially salad dressings. Either peel them and enjoy whole or try the Citrus Fennel Salad with Toasted Sunflower Seeds on page 184.

Important note: The compounds in grapefruit can increase circulating levels of several prescription drugs, including statins. This means that the risk of muscle toxicity associated with statins may increase when you eat grapefruit, so check with your doctor if you're on prescription medications before chowing down on grapefruit.

HEMP SEEDS

Also known as hemp hearts, these soft, nutty seeds with the shell removed taste like a cross between a pine nut and a sunflower seed. They are so versatile in raw recipes, and although small, they are mighty nutritional powerhouses. They are not a crop that attracts a lot of pests, making it unnecessary to purchase them certified organic if your budget does not allow this. Plus, they're a Canadian crop, from the Prairies!

Joyous Detox facts about hemp seeds

- Benefit cells. An excellent source of omega-3 fatty acids, which are important to reduce inflammation and keep your cells healthy.
- Plant protein. A fantastic source of easily digestible plant-based protein. In fact, hemp seeds contain all the essential amino acids.
- Good fats. With their healthy fats and plant-based protein, they keep you feeling fuller longer. They are also a great source of a type of fat called GLA, which is essential for healthy hair, skin and nails.

How to enjoy them: Sprinkle hemp hearts on just about anything, from salads to soups and smoothies. They add the perfect creaminess to the Best Ever Hemp Caesar Salad Dressing on page 199 and boost up the protein in the Energy Booster Balls on page 181.

HERBS

Fresh herbs are easily added to just about any recipe, whether it calls for them or not. They are one of the best nutrition bangs for your buck, especially if you grow them on your windowsill. Here are some of my favourite herbs to use both for taste and nutritional benefits.

Parsley

- **Nutrient-dense.** A nutrient powerhouse, containing vitamins A, B, C and K and the minerals iron and potassium. It also contains detoxifying chlorophyll (anything green contains chlorophyll).
- **Anti-inflammatory.** Contains the volatile oil eugenol, which provides anti-inflammatory benefits.
- **Cleansing.** Known to help stimulate bowel function, and it is blood cleansing.

Basil

- **Protection from toxins.** Full of water-soluble flavonoids that protect cell structures and chromosomes from radiation and the oxygen-based damage that toxins can cause.
- **Natural antibiotic.** Contains antibacterial volatile oils.
- **Anti-inflammatory.** Contains eugenol, which inhibits the enzyme cyclo-oxygenase (the same enzyme inhibited by NSAIDs).
- **Rich in antioxidants.** A very good source of antioxidant carotenoids and vitamin C.
- **Good fats.** A good plant-based source of omega-3 essential fatty acids.

Cilantro

- **Rich in antioxidants.** Contains a wide range of antioxidant phytonutrients, including many carotenoids.
- **Natural antibiotic.** Contains a powerful antimicrobial compound that may help prevent food-borne illnesses such as salmonella.
- **Benefits cells.** The seeds (coriander) may help reduce the amount of damaged fats in animal cell membranes and lower total levels of LDL ("bad" cholesterol) while increasing HDL ("good" cholesterol).

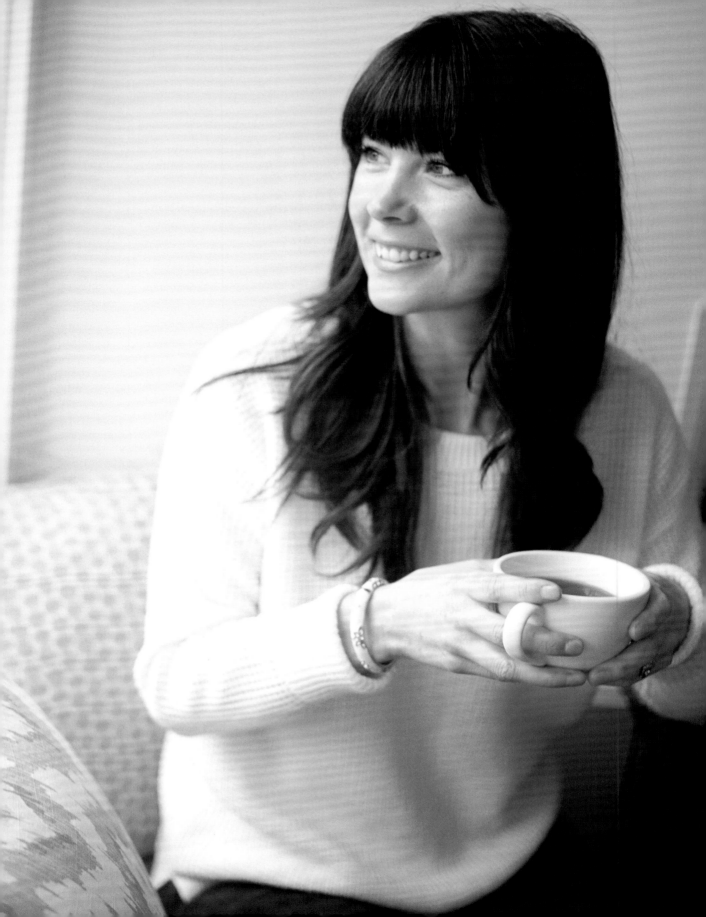

Mint

- Digestion friendly. Has the ability to relax smooth muscle, which can help alleviate the symptoms of irritable bowel syndrome, dyspepsia and indigestion.
- Cancer prevention. Contains phytonutrients that have been shown in animal studies to possibly help stop the growth of pancreatic, mammary and liver tumours, as well as protect against cancer formation in the colon, skin and lungs.
- Natural antibiotic and antifungal.

LEGUMES

Black beans, adzuki beans, chickpeas, navy beans, lentils . . . the list goes on and on. Legumes are a favourite of vegans and vegetarians, but no matter your dietary preferences, they should be a regular feature on your dinner plate because of their broad range of nutrients.

Joyous Detox facts about legumes

- Cancer fighter. Contain a wide range of cancer-preventative phyto-nutrients, including isoflavones and phytosterols.
- Rich in fibre. Legumes are loaded with high levels of soluble fibre that helps lower cholesterol, balance blood sugar and cleanse the intestines.
- Aid blood sugar balance. Contain a balance of complex carbohydrates and protein that provides a slow, steady source of glucose.
- Aid healthy cholesterol levels. Even more effective than whole grains at lowering LDL ("bad" cholesterol) and triglycerides.

How to enjoy them: The roasted chickpeas done three different ways are the perfect crunchy snack (pages 171–173), and the three mason jar salads (pages 188–191) are both nourishing and fulfilling recipes as a main event of a meal.

LEMONS (AND LIMES)

You've likely heard about the benefits of lemon and water. I've been singing its praises for years on my blog, *Joyous Health*, and at every workshop I teach. Lemon juice is fresh, bright and uplifting, with liver-loving benefits.

Joyous Detox facts about lemons

- Digestion friendly. Aid digestion by increasing saliva flow (the first stage of digestion) and stomach acid production, as well as stimulating bowel movements, reducing constipation and alleviating flatulence and bloating.
- Liver lover. Benefit the liver by encouraging the formation of bile, which carries toxins away from the liver.
- Rich in vitamin C. One of the most important antioxidants in nature neutralizes free radicals in the body.
- Cancer fighter. Lemons have been shown to help fight cancer of the mouth, skin, lung, breast, stomach and colon with the help of compounds called limonoids, which are present in citrus.

How to enjoy them: The most joyous way to start the day, and my favourite detox habit, is drinking freshly squeezed lemon with water first thing in the morning.

Important Note: Do not drink lemon and water if you have stomach ulcers.

MATCHA GREEN TEA

Matcha literally means "powdered tea." It is essentially ground tea leaves, whereas green tea is simply brewed leaves. It is more nutrient-dense than green tea because you are consuming the whole leaf rather than just steeping the leaves. My favourite ways to enjoy matcha are either in a smoothie or in a latte made with coconut milk and raw honey. Matcha is an acquired taste, and many people dislike it at first. However, if you combine it with other ingredients (don't worry, no one will scold you for not being a purist), it takes the edge off and may make it more enjoyable for you.

Joyous Detox facts about matcha

- **Energizing.** Matcha provides what I call a "clean energy" because even though it contains nearly three times as much caffeine as green tea, it also contains a naturally calming amino acid, L-theanine, which is helpful if you plan on eliminating coffee while detoxing.
- **Aids detox.** Boosts the production of groups of detoxification enzymes that use catechin bioflavonoids to convert carcinogens into harmless chemicals. Also extremely rich in chlorophyll, making it a superior beverage for detoxification.
- **Antioxidant-rich.** Packed with antioxidants, including the powerful EGCG, which supports cardiovascular health and metabolism.

How to enjoy it: The simplest way to enjoy matcha is simply to brew a cup of this antioxidant powerhouse or make the Matcha Green Tea Smoothie on page 145.

OATS

Oats are a wonderful grain that add substance and nourishment to any recipe. They are naturally gluten-free, but if you have celiac disease then you may want to buy "certified gluten-free" oats to ensure there is no cross-contamination with gluten. My favourite time of year to eat oatmeal is in the winter because it's the quintessential comfort food. Oats are a detox superfood, fantastic for diabetics (they help regulate blood sugar) and heart-healthy (they help reduce inflammation).

Joyous Detox facts about oats

- **Fibre-rich.** Oats are high in both soluble and insoluble fibre, which keeps you satiated and keeps your digestive system moving and eliminating effectively. They contain a specific type of fibre known as beta-glucan that has an extra-beneficial effect on cholesterol levels.
- **Immune booster.** Beta-glucan helps neutrophils (the most abundant type of nonspecific immune cell) navigate to the site of an infection more quickly and enhance their ability to eliminate the bacteria they find there.

- Antioxidants. Antioxidant compounds called avenanthramides, found mainly in oats, help prevent free radicals from damaging LDL cholesterol.

How to enjoy them: Overnight Oatmeal with Peaches and Apricots on page 123 and Strawberry Oat Mini Pancakes on page 103 are both delicious ways to incorporate oats into your diet.

ONIONS

Onions have a bad rep because of the smell they leave on your breath. But this smell is a telltale sign of the onion's detox power. Just eat some parsley (also a detox superfood!) afterward to neutralize the smell.

Joyous Detox facts about onions

- Detox support. Contain sulphur compounds that support detoxification pathways and protect the liver. Sulphur also helps the body to detox from heavy metals like lead, arsenic and cadmium.
- Antibacterial. These sulphur-containing compounds and the flavonoid quercetin have been shown to help prevent bacterial infection.
- Anti-inflammatory. A rich source of quercetin, a powerful antioxidant flavonoid that has a broad range of benefits, from reducing inflammation to reducing the risk of certain cancers.

How to enjoy them: Onions are in dozens of recipes in *Joyous Detox* because they pack a lot of flavour and detox benefits. Enjoy them in Chickpea Blender Soup on page 161, Warm Sweet Potato Kale Bowl with Quinoa on page 213 or Rainbow Mason Jar Salad on page 188.

QUINOA

Quinoa is one of my favourite plant-based sources of protein. It is an incredibly versatile food because it takes on the flavour of whatever you cook it with. You can enjoy it sweet or savoury, cooked or sprouted, cold or hot, and it is filling and delicious. Quinoa is gluten-free, making it the perfect pseudo-grain to accompany any recipe.

Joyous Detox facts about quinoa

- **Complete protein.** It is a complete plant-based protein and high in the amino acid lysine, which is involved in tissue repair.
- **Antioxidant-rich.** Contains significant amounts of such antioxidants as ferulic, coumaric, hydroxybenzoic and vanillic acid.
- **High in fibre.** A good source of fibre, which promotes the elimination of waste.
- **Anti-inflammatory.** Has a diverse range of anti-inflammatory nutrients, including omega-3 fatty acids, which help your cells to be more permeable so they can more effectively release toxins; are needed for all liver functions, including detoxification; and can help counter toxin-induced inflammation in the body.

How to enjoy it: Quinoa takes on the flavour of the other ingredients, making it a very versatile grain. It is also a great substitute for oats. These recipes are wonderfully fulfilling: Sesame Orange Quinoa Bowl on page 230 and Salmon Quinoa Cakes with Lemon Sauce on page 229.

SEA VEGETABLES

Sea veggies were completely foreign to me until I became a nutritionist and learned about all their health benefits. From kelp to arame, nori to dulse and kombu, these salty and delicious foods are the perfect addition to any wrap, salad or soup. I even love eating roasted seaweed snacks straight out of the bag!

Joyous Detox facts about sea veggies

- **Antioxidant-rich.** Contain powerful antioxidants that help to alkalize the blood and strengthen the digestive tract.
- **Aid detox.** The algin in sea veggies absorbs toxins from the digestive tract in much the same way a water softener removes the hardness from tap water. It can also bind to radioactive waste in the body so it can be removed.
- **Mineral-rich.** Sea veggies offer the broadest range of minerals of any food, containing virtually all the minerals found in the ocean—the same minerals that are found in human blood.

How to enjoy them: I mix sea veggies into salads and add them to soups to increase the mineral content. Cooking beans with kombu is a great way to reduce the gassiness associated with beans.

SUNFLOWER SEEDS

Even though I also love pumpkin seeds for detox, I find that people overlook the humble but equally powerful sunflower seed. Be sure to purchase unsalted, unroasted seeds to maximize the health benefits.

Joyous Detox facts about sunflower seeds

- **Liver lover.** High in selenium and vitamin E, both of which are important for detoxification of the liver.
- **Digestion friendly.** Easily digested protein and a source of good fat.
- **Heart-healthy.** They help prevent cholesterol building up in the arteries.

How to enjoy them: Seeds are a wonderful alternative if you have nut allergies. No-Bake Superfood Breakfast Bars on page 119 really fill the hunger gap in the morning, and the Black Rice Butternut Squash Salad on page 187 is a fulfilling side or main dish. Sunflower seeds can be ground into a dip for a wonderful substitute for hummus; try the Sunny Punchy Seed Spread on page 198.

TURMERIC

This beautiful mustard-yellow spice is one of the best liver-detoxifying spices available. It gives curry its rich yellow colour, but not its flavour. It's actually quite mild. Before it's transformed into a powder, it starts out as a root—part of the ginger family. I buy organic turmeric powder because the root can be tough to find at grocery stores.

Joyous Detox facts about turmeric

- **Powerful plant chemical.** Its active component, a powerful plant chemical called curcumin, contains all the medicinal benefits (see next page).

- Liver lover. Stimulates the production of bile, which aids in the elimination of toxins from the liver.
- Nutrient-dense. Contains a variety of minerals, including calcium, potassium and magnesium.
- Anti-inflammatory. Has been shown to be an anti-inflammatory superfood with effects comparable to drugs such as hydrocortisone and phenylbutazone as well as over-the-counter drugs such as Motrin. Eating a whole food has no side effects, unlike pharmaceutical drugs. Hurray for real food!

How to enjoy it: Try the Daily Detox Zinger Elixir on page 135 and the Soothing Golden Smoothie on page 144. Turmeric is a mild spice and can be added to many recipes.

Joyous Affirmation

I choose food that nourishes my body, mind and soul.

3

DETOX
LIFESTYLE HABITS

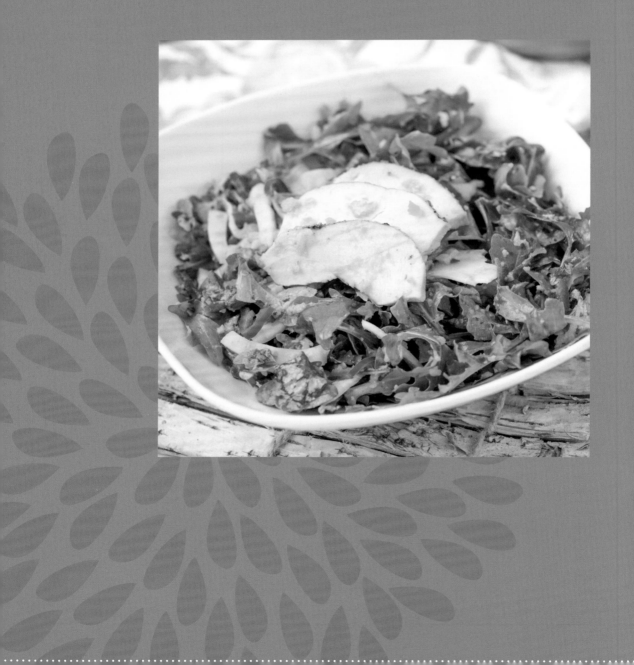

Now that you know all the detox superfoods to stock in your kitchen and their health benefits, let's talk about lifestyle habits that help detoxification. These habits are just as important as eating detox foods and have similar benefits that range from improved digestion to weight loss and glowing skin!

I recommend you try a new detox habit each week and keep doing the ones you enjoy the most. Dry skin brushing is a detox habit I make time for every single day because it really does make my skin glow. So do yoga and powerwalking. And of course these habits have more benefits than just detoxification.

If you feel that you don't have time to implement any new health habits, think of it this way: making time for these detox lifestyle habits means that you are taking time for self-care. You *deserve* self-care. When we take better care of ourselves, we are kinder to others, we are more productive at work and our overall happiness improves dramatically.

DRINK PLENTY OF WATER

Did you know your body is 60 percent water? Your brain and heart are 70 percent water, and your lungs are just over 80 percent water. Your skin is 64 percent water, which is why drinking water is beautifying! Yet I know from reviewing hundreds of people's food journals that this simple habit is probably the most overlooked.

Water is necessary for every single metabolic process in the body and vital to the life of every cell. It is absolutely essential for detoxification to occur, because a dehydrated body cannot effectively eliminate stored toxins or fat. Water also helps deliver nutrients to the cells and remove waste via the urine. It also cleanses your kidneys, allowing them to function optimally.

Water should be the first thing that your lips touch in the morning, not coffee or food.

We hear a lot of different advice about how much water we're supposed to drink. There are formulas based on your weight and height, but I actually don't agree with this method of calculation because it doesn't take into account many factors, such as your caffeine consumption, how much you're sweating or how many cooked versus raw foods you eat.

I recommend you drink six to twelve 8-ounce (250 mL) glasses of water each day. You can determine your water needs based on the colour of your urine, how thirsty you are and the above-mentioned factors (caffeine, sweating, cooked/raw foods). If you're drinking enough water, your urine should be a pale yellow.

Keep in mind that you can drink *too much* water, which puts extra strain on your kidneys. While this is rare, if your urine is always clear, then you are drinking too much water.

One way to increase your hydration level beyond simply drinking water is to consume more raw fruits and vegetables, soups and herbal teas.

As for the type of water you drink, tap water (depending where you live) is likely the safest bet, provided you use a water filter to remove the heavy metals. A basic carbon filter will remove most of the toxins, such as arsenic, lead and cadmium, and help get rid of the chlorine taste. Even though most tap water is considered safe, many public water supplies in North America still contain traces of pharmaceutical drugs, pesticides and other industrial chemicals. If you wish to drink water without any such toxic elements, including fluoride, you will need to drink distilled or reverse osmosis water. Alternatively, you can look for fresh spring water directly from Mama Nature, but you drink this water at your own risk, as it could be contaminated with agricultural chemicals from nearby farms.

DRINK LEMON AND WATER OR APPLE CIDER VINEGAR AND WATER

I have written about this extensively in my first book, *Joyous Health*, and have videos on my YouTube channel about this essential detox habit. Whether you are detoxing or not, I recommend you drink water with lemon or apple cider vinegar every single morning on an empty stomach—before eating or drinking anything else. This is one of the simplest and most effective daily cleansing rituals you can do for your body.

How to

1. Add fresh juice from ¼ to ½ a lemon or 1 tsp (5 mL) unpasteurized apple cider vinegar to a 2-cup (500 mL) glass of room-temperature filtered water. Drink every single morning on an empty stomach, before food.

Benefits

- Stimulates the liver to produce bile, a carrier of toxins
- Enhances digestion by stimulating digestive secretions and reducing bloating
- Stimulates the liver's detoxifying enzymes
- Lemon juice is a good source of vitamin C, which protects the liver
- Results in glowing skin and whiter whites of the eyes
- Allows better bowel movements
- Reduces heartburn

Many people are concerned that lemon will wear down the enamel of their teeth. If this is a concern for you, use a straw or simply swish plain water in your mouth after drinking lemon and water. If drinking lemon and water makes you feel ill, causes canker sores or gives you digestive problems, you may have a citrus sensitivity, so switch to apple cider vinegar and water.

SWEATING

I don't think I've ever left a sauna or a yoga session without noticing that my skin was glowing! When you sweat, your body releases excess water, minerals and salts. Deep sweating, such as in a sauna or during hot yoga, may help remove waste products from the body, including heavy metals and unwanted chemicals, as well as aid in fat loss. This is why you must drink plenty of fresh, filtered water every day.

Infrared saunas are the best way to get a relaxing, deep sweat to enhance detoxification and improve the health of your body. They work differently than a traditional sauna, heating the body rather than the air. Not only do these saunas increase sweating but they also boost circulation, which, in turn, increases the removal of toxins via the liver.

Hot yoga is another easy method to get sweating. Just be sure that while you are following the detox meal plan in this book, you feel energetic enough for an invigorating yoga class.

If you have high blood pressure or vertigo, or are pregnant, being in a sauna is not recommended. Be sure to speak to your healthcare practitioner.

DETOX BATH

Having a footbath or a whole body bath in Epsom salts (magnesium sulphate) is a popular detox habit nowadays, even though it is an ancient method of detoxification. Not only can it assist your body in eliminating toxins but it is also incredibly relaxing and puts you in a "chilled out" state of mind that allows detoxification to happen with ease.

When you have an Epsom salt bath, you absorb magnesium through the skin. This is a good thing because, according to Dr. Carolyn Dean, author of *The Magnesium Miracle*, magnesium is required for more than 325 enzymes to work properly and helps keep toxins out of the brain. Magnesium is essential for bone, heart and brain health because it works in concert with calcium. Many health conditions, including anxiety, osteoporosis and heart disease, can result if you are deficient in this important mineral.

How to

1. Make sure you have enough time in your schedule to enjoy the bath and don't feel rushed. I recommend doing it before bed for about 45 minutes, then go to sleep right after.

2. Fill your bathtub with warm water, not scalding hot, which would be too drying to the skin and could elevate your body temperature and heart rate, preventing you from relaxing.
3. Add 2 cups (500 mL) of food-grade Epsom salts to the water.
4. Optional: For extra relaxation, add a few drops of your favourite organic essential oil to the water. My favourite essential oil for relaxation is lavender.

DRY SKIN BRUSHING

Dry skin brushing is an inexpensive and simple detox habit that I do every single day. I've been singing its praises for as long as I can remember, and I talked about it in my first book, *Joyous Health*. Dry skin brushing has been practised for centuries around the world, including in Russia, Scandinavia and India. It makes perfect sense to dry skin brush when you consider that your skin is an organ of elimination.

> ### Joyous Tip
> • • •
> Keeping your pores free of dead skin cells that would otherwise result in dull, dry skin helps your skin better regenerate and allows toxins to be eliminated through the skin when you sweat.

Benefits

- Stimulates the lymphatic system, a network of vessels that actually holds a larger amount of fluid than your circulatory system. Improving the flow of lymph fluid assists in the removal of waste products from the body and enhances detoxification.
- Increases circulation, which gets your blood flowing and prevents stagnation of fluids in the body
- Removes dead skin cells and allows the skin to glow
- Improves skin texture and makes skin softer
- May decrease cellulite
- Is incredibly energizing and invigorating

How to

1. Choose a natural-bristle body brush with fairly stiff bristles that are comfortably uncomfortable but do not scratch your skin.
2. Dry brush before every shower.
3. Using a light amount of pressure, move the brush in small, circular motions toward the heart. Start with your feet and work your way up to your neck. Do not dry brush your face or your nipples, or any area that is sensitive or inflamed.
4. When you reach your breasts, brush toward your armpits to stimulate lymphatic drainage of your breasts. Be sure to spend a little more time where you have lymph nodes—the back of your knees, your groin, your tummy, inside your elbows, your armpits and your neck.
5. Say or think loving thoughts about every part of your body as you dry skin brush.
6. Shower after you have dry skin brushed your whole body.
7. Do this four to seven times a week. Once you've nailed down the routine, you'll be able to do it in less than 5 minutes.

You can buy a dry skin brush at the health food store.

ALTERNATING WARM/COLD SHOWER

The first time I went to a spa where they recommended I relax in the hot tub and then plunge into an ice-cold bath for a few minutes, I thought they were completely nuts . . . until I tried it! Going from a warm shower to a freezing-cold one might sound rather unpleasant, but once you've done it a few times you'll be totally addicted. It's invigorating and energy boosting!

> ### *Joyous Tip*
> • • •
> Avoid hot showers. They strip away your skin's natural oils, leading to dry, dull, lifeless skin. Warm and cold showers help your skin glow!

Benefits

- Improves circulation, which enhances the removal and elimination of waste and gives your skin a healthy glow
- May stimulate weight loss. One study found that being exposed to extremely cold temperatures increased brown fat activity fifteenfold. That translates to losing up to nine pounds a year. Toxins are fat-soluble, so when you lose fat, you also detoxify.
- May help relieve depression. Your skin has more cold receptors than warm ones, so exposure to cold water sends a massive amount of electrical impulses to the brain. Research suggests this brain stimulation may have an antidepressant effect.
- Increases blood flow, which in turn increases energy and alertness.

How to

1. Start out with a warm shower for 2 minutes. Change the temperature to as cold as it will go, and shower for 1 minute.
2. Alternate back and forth three or four times.
3. Alternatively, start your shower cold for 2 to 3 minutes and then gradually increase the temperature until it's comfortable for the rest of your shower.

POWERWALKING

Regular exercise is essential for detoxification, for lymph drainage and to prevent stagnating energy in your body. When your heart rate increases, so does circulation and the flow of lymph fluid. This increase in circulation enhances digestion, relieves stress and gets toxins flowing out of your body to reduce your overall toxic load.

I recommend powerwalking for 30 to 45 minutes every single day whether you are detoxing or not. Too many of us sit around for six to eight hours a day. A sedentary lifestyle puts you at a greater risk for obesity and heart disease, according to the *British Journal of Sports Medicine.*

And you can increase the health benefits by walking outside in nature. Being outside in nature actually lights up areas of the brain associated with love, empathy and happiness. Nature and greenspace are like a vitamin—I call it vitamin G. Take advantage of this free vitamin every single day you can!

DIGITAL DETOX

When was the last time you disconnected from social media for 24 hours, or a whole weekend? If you've never considered this type of detox, then maybe it's time you tried it out. Taking deliberate time out and disconnecting from all things digital is a deeply rewarding experience. You will find you become more creative and productive. You will find that your relationships improve, and you will realize that it's more important to connect with people instead of things. It's a good way to remind yourself of what *really* matters.

Research shows that the average person spends more than six hours a day exposed to screens on smartphones, computers and televisions. Just look at the number of people staring down at their phones while they walk down the street. We are more connected to our phones than we are to other human beings! How often do you see a couple in a restaurant having a relationship with their phones instead of with each other? This excessive screen time is associated with psychological difficulties, including anxiety and depression, according to a study published in *Preventative Medicine*. Another consideration is the increase in radiation we are now exposed to from constantly being connected.

Work obligations can make it challenging to completely disconnect—I can relate! However, my husband and I do a weekend digital detox a few times a year. When we are back at the office on Monday morning we always feel more rejuvenated. Vacations are a great time to do a digital detox as well. I highly recommend it!

How to

1. Choose a specific time frame during which you will disconnect. Make sure it's at least 24 hours. A weekend or vacation is a great time to do this.
2. For this time period, avoid using any mobile device, smartphone, tablet or computer.

Beyond a time-limited digital detox, I also suggest you consider an evening digital detox every day. That's right—*every day*. Disconnect from your devices when you get home from work or at a specific time each day. You will find this allows you to better connect with yourself and others. If you live with someone or have children, I recommend that you do the digital detox together.

MASSAGE THERAPY

We all know how good we feel after a session of massage therapy, and it's not only because we're incredibly relaxed. Massage therapy helps enhance detoxification and stimulates the lymphatic system to function optimally.

Your body is under physical and mental stress 24/7, and this stress causes it to build up metabolites, by-products that naturally occur from metabolic processes. Massage therapy is the manipulation of soft tissue in order to increase circulation (assuming you are having a full-body massage), according to registered massage therapist Phil Teno.

The increased circulation that results from having a massage helps to flush out metabolites and toxic waste naturally through perspiration, urination and bowel movements. According to Teno, specific techniques on the abdomen and large intestine can stimulate this process, as well as help with regularity by reducing constipation and toxic buildup. Massage therapists sometimes use dry skin brushing along with a lymphatic massage to stimulate lymphatic drainage and further aid in the removal of toxins and waste products from the body.

If your budget and time allow, I recommend a massage with a registered massage therapist once or twice a month. If your health benefits cover massage therapy, then definitely take advantage of it for the detoxification benefits!

MEDITATION

The National Science Foundation estimated that we can have up to fifty thousand thoughts a day, and even more if you are a deep thinker. Unfortunately, it's estimated that close to three-quarters of these thoughts can be negative or just pure nonsense (although there's nothing wrong with the latter, in my opinion—sometimes the best ideas come out of nonsense thoughts). Giving your brain a break and allowing it to relax is a great idea, especially if you are one of those with a "monkey brain."

I interviewed Christine Russell, co-founder of 889 Yoga in Toronto, on the topic of meditation because she's an expert! Here's what she had to say about meditation.

For the body, meditation is a great way to detox. In meditation the body is given a chance to rest and relax. Meditation frees up red blood cells and lets us heal our nervous system. When stressed or angry, for example, cortisol, a stress hormone, stays in our bodies for 24 hours. Meditation counteracts this. It acts to calm the body, and helps us to remember how to find this calm when our bodies need it. Meditation provides us the opportunity to awaken the nervous system so it works for us when we need it: it helps our bodies slow down so that when life's challenges present themselves to us, we are prepared and we are not fighting. Our bodies need this regular exposure to stillness and introspection so that the body can work optimally for us!

For me, meditation makes space psychologically in my life. It cleanses my mind and body, and it makes new architecture in the parts of our mind and body for peace and calm. It's important to note that meditation is not a cure-all for all the difficulties in your life. I wish! What a meditation practice does is give you the tools to handle these difficult situations with more ease and grace. It helps me to react less and respond more thoughtfully. It helps me to shift my thoughts quicker when they go south. It helps me to be more compassionate toward others because I have cleared out and cultivated space to be more compassionate toward myself.

Christine also shared a quick how-to guide for meditation whether you are a newbie or not.

How much time: Set aside 5 minutes every morning (and 5 minutes each night if you can!).

Where: Find a cozy spot in your home without distractions and without technology. If you want to go one step further, you can create a very simple altar for yourself by adding a few meaningful things to your space. They could be a card someone gave you, an inspirational image, a crystal, a Buddha, anything you want!

What you need: A cushion to sit on, two small pillows for under your knees and a timer.

How: Sit cross-legged on the cushion so that your hips are above your knees. You want to sit on the edge of the cushion, not the middle of it. Place two small pillows or towels under your knees for support. With a straight spine, rest your hands on your knees—palms up if you want to be energized, palms down if you feel you need grounding.

Time: Set your timer for 5 minutes. If you are using your smartphone, turn it to airplane mode so there are no electromagnetic waves in your space and no "dings" distracting you.

HOW TO MEDITATE

1. Take three deep breaths in through your nose and sigh out loud out your mouth.

2. Begin gentle, natural breathing in and out of your nose.

3. Tune in to your breath in and out of your nose.

4. Imagine you are tracing your breath from the tip of your nostril up to your third eye point, just between your two eyes. Exhale to release.

5. Repeat this breath tracing for 5 minutes.

6. Bring your hands crossed one on top of the other onto your heart, or bring your hands together in prayer, and repeat the following: May I be peaceful, may I be at ease, may I be filled with loving-kindness, may I be free. May all beings be peaceful, may all beings be at ease, may all beings be filled with loving-kindness, may all beings be free.

7. Open your eyes. Give thanks for something and share a prayer for the highest good.

PERSONAL CARE DETOX

Unfortunately, in Canada and the United States, the personal care industry still has a long way to go when it comes to cleaning up the ingredients in personal care products. The majority of products on the market today contain a whole plethora of cancer-causing, hormone-disrupting and allergy-inducing substances. It is up to you, as a consumer, to take charge of your health, be informed and avoid products that contain these harmful chemicals.

Clean, toxin-free and safe personal care products are something I'm fiercely committed to for the health of both my family and my planet. We are so fortunate that clean and safe products that *actually* work are now available in abundance at retail stores. And if you're not near a store that sells them, you can purchase products online.

You can benefit from a personal care detox because you'll reduce your daily toxic load of hormone-disrupting ingredients, carcinogens, neurotoxins and more. You will likely find that eliminating unnecessary chemicals in your personal care products improves your hormonal health, your skin and your digestion.

Some experts might argue that it's the dose that makes the poison, and microscopic amounts of estrogen-mimicking chemicals in your shampoo won't affect you. Oh, but they do! These so-called experts fail to consider the multiple products the average person uses every day with literally hundreds of chemicals in them. Even if you use only a small handful of products with hormone-disrupting ingredients, these chemicals build up in your already burdened body and accumulate in your fatty tissues. A microscopic dose in one product multiplied by a dozen or more products used each day for months and years is no longer a microscopic amount.

And what about young children, pregnant and breastfeeding women and those who are immune-compromised? They are at an even greater risk of being affected by chemicals in personal care products. And let's not forget the environmental reasons to avoid these chemicals: they go down our drains and end up in our lakes and rivers, harming aquatic life. Do you need any more reasons to ditch the chemical-laden personal care products in favour of safe products?

Environmental Defence, Canada's most effective environmental action organization, publishes a list of the top ten ingredients to avoid in personal care products. I recommend that you do a personal care detox as soon as you can! Review all the lotions, potions and bottles you use, from toothpaste to mascara to body wash and lip gloss, and make sure they do not contain any of the Toxic Ten, as determined by Environmental Defence.

Getting your partner or family on board can sometimes be challenging, but if you start changing over your products slowly, they might not even notice!

TOXIC TEN INGREDIENTS

1,4-DIOXANE A probable carcinogen and an eye and respiratory tract irritant found in trace amounts in some cosmetics, personal care and cleaning products. It doesn't appear on product labels because it's a contaminant created during the manufacturing process. Instead, watch the label for sodium laureth sulphate (SLES), a petroleum-based ingredient that acts as a foaming agent. SLES can be contaminated with 1,4-dioxane. Additionally, check product labels for "PEG compounds" and chemicals that include "xynol," "ceteareth" and "oleth" in their names.

ARTIFICIAL MUSKS Hormone-disrupting chemicals that are often included in fragrance or parfum. Fragrance chemicals often contain endocrine-disrupting phthalates and are linked to allergies, immune system toxicity, headaches and dizziness. Watch out for "fragrance," "parfum" or "musk" in the ingredient list of personal care products.

BHA and BHT Butylated hydroxyanisole and butylated hydroxytoluene are synthetic antioxidants that are used as preservatives in personal care products and cosmetics. Studies show these chemicals are carcinogenic, endocrine disrupting and allergenic. BHA and BHT can be found in personal care products, including lipstick, eyeshadow, concealer and moisturizers.

COAL TAR–DERIVED COLOURS Associated with non-Hodgkin's lymphoma, multiple myeloma, acute leukemia, bladder cancer, contact dermatitis and severe facial edema. In the short term, common reactions are itching, burning, hives and blistering of the skin. Coal tar–derived colours, including P-phenylenediamine (PPD, or paraphenylenediamine), are often used in permanent hair dyes, with higher concentration in darker shades.

FORMALDEHYDE-RELEASING AGENTS Chemicals that slowly off-gas formaldehyde throughout their life, to be inhaled by the user of the product. There are many health concerns about formaldehyde because it is an immune system toxin, a skin irritant and a known carcinogen. Chemicals that release formaldehyde are found in hair care products, hair colouring, nail products and many other beauty products. They may appear as any of the following on a label: DMDM hydantoin, diazolidinyl urea, imidazolidinyl urea, methenamine, quaternium-15 and sodium hydroxymethylglycinate.

PARABENS The most commonly used preservatives in cosmetics and are often used as unlisted fragrance ingredients. They are absorbed through the skin and go straight into the bloodstream and organs. Parabens are linked to endocrine disruption, reproductive toxicity, immunotoxicity, neurotoxicity and skin irritation. They are also linked to breast cancer. Parabens are found in a number of personal care products, including shampoo, moisturizer, shaving cream, cleansing gels, personal lubricant, deodorant and toothpaste.

PETROLATUM Commonly known as petroleum jelly, a virtually odourless and tasteless gel that helps to smooth and soften skin. It has been associated with cancer, skin irritations and allergies. Petrolatum can be found in skin creams, wax depilatories, eyebrow pencils, eyeshadows, lipsticks, conditioner and blush.

PHTHALATES Man-made chemicals used as plasticizers and as preservatives for fragrance. Research has shown that phthalates disrupt hormones and can cause birth defects of the male reproductive organs. They are also persistent in the environment. You'll find phthalates in many cosmetic and personal care products, including scented items and nail products.

SILICONE CHEMICALS Also known as siloxanes, detrimental to the environment and have raised concerns for their effects on human health. Absorbed through the skin, siloxanes can contribute to skin irritation and have been linked to cancer. They are used in a variety of hair products, as well as eye and face makeup, manicuring preparations, skin creams and oils, and foot powders and sprays.

TRICLOSAN A synthetic antibacterial/antifungal agent that has been linked to superbugs and is toxic to the environment. Triclosan is used in a wide variety of personal care products, including shaving creams, hair conditioners, deodorants, liquid soaps, hand soaps, facial cleansers and disinfectants. Watch out for products that are marketed as "antibacterial" or contain the name "Microban," such as hand sanitizer, lotion and toothpaste.

Source: EnvironmentalDefence.ca

1. **Be an avid label reader.** You already know the importance of reading food labels; the same goes for reading labels on personal care products. Avoidance is the best way to get these chemicals out of your home and away from your body. Don't buy any products with any of the "Toxic Ten" ingredients listed in the chart on page 57. Reading labels may not protect you 100 percent from harmful chemicals because companies do not always disclose everything, but avoiding what you do see on a label is a good start.

2. **Be a DIY diva.** I personally love making my own products, from body scrubs to moisturizers. I know exactly what ingredients are going into them, and each one has a purpose. Some of my favourite DIY ingredients are sweet almond oil, witch hazel, coconut oil and organic essential oils. Additionally, you can make an amazing hydrating facial mask out of ingredients in your kitchen such as raw cacao, avocado and honey. You can find plenty of free beauty DIY recipes on my blog; check out the "Beauty" section.

3. **Don't wear perfume, cologne or any fragranced body spray.** The problem with fragrance is that, under a patent rights loophole, companies do not have to disclose all the ingredients and can hide hundreds of chemicals under the terms "parfum" and "fragrance." Products with added fragrance and commercial fragrance products

Clean up your clothing

A popular video I posted on my YouTube channel a couple of years ago was "10 Ways to Have Less Waste." The two most important points in that video were "buy less" and "buy quality." While I was doing research for that video, I discovered that North Americans purchase clothing to excess. In fact, the average person buys sixty-eight pieces of clothing and seven pairs of shoes each year, according to Elizabeth Cline, author of *Overdressed: The Shockingly High Cost of Cheap Fashion.* Clothing has become so cheap that many people consider it disposable.

But this cheap clothing has a dirty secret. Have you ever given that new twenty-dollar shirt a sniff? Much of the cheap clothing is produced in developing countries (likely by labourers who are not paid fairly) and shipped overseas after being treated with horrendous chemicals such as formaldehyde (to prevent can contain many hidden ingredients that are hormone disrupters, carcinogens and allergens. Ever wondered why you get a headache from your co-worker's perfume? Instead, use organic essential oils diluted in sweet almond oil.

4. **Don't dye your hair.** It's a fairly well-known fact that hair dyes have been linked to bladder cancer because they contain carcinogenic chemicals. Most of these dyes contain coal tar–derived colours, which are best avoided. Simply ask your stylist to use a clean hair dye product or go to a green beauty spa that uses toxin-free hair dyes.

5. **Use a safer nail polish.** If you're like me, you like to have painted nails. The best part is it's not hard to find great colours that are "three-free," which means they do not contain dibutyl phthalate, formaldehyde or toluene, the three worst chemicals in many nail polishes. You can also find "five-free," meaning the product is also free of the allergens camphor and formaldehyde resin. All these ingredients could do everything from disrupt your endocrine system to cause cancer. Some great brands are butter London, Zoya, RGB and Suncoat.

6. **Choose fruit-pigmented makeup.** Heavy metals are abundant in cosmetics. They're what make your lipstick that perfect ruby red. The majority of cosmetics are contaminated with lead, cadmium and mercury. The scary part is that companies do not have to disclose these ingredients, which are toxic to the nervous system. While the amount in one smear of lipstick might be less than the amount you get in your drinking water, it's the daily use that adds up. Some great brands that are free of heavy metals include 100% Pure, W3LL People and RMS.

mildew during shipping), harmful dyes, phthalates and more. In fact, up to two thousand chemicals are used in the processing of fabrics, some of which are known to cause skin irritation, asthma and even cancer.

Unfortunately, it's almost impossible to know whether an item of clothing you are purchasing has been treated with toxic chemicals. However, some key phrases on a tag indicate the use of chemicals: "pre-shrunk," "fire-retardant," "stain-resistant," "moth-repellant" and "no-iron." If you see any of these on the label, leave them on the rack. These types of fabrics use a chemical called PBDE that accumulates in fatty tissues. The U.S. Environmental Protection Agency has advised that chemicals used to achieve the "no-iron" properties of a garment are known as perfluorinated chemicals, and they have been associated with an increase in certain cancers.

As you can see, your body has a lot of chemicals to contend with, not just from food but from toxins in clothing as well. Consider taking a break from purchasing new clothes for a while, and when you do need something new, before you purchase it consider where it's from and what it might have been treated with.

Sleeping

It's no secret that eating well and exercising are essential for preventing disease, promoting well-being and enhancing detoxification. However, one overlooked habit that is equally important is adequate sleep. In my own clinical practice, clients who get everything right except making sleep a priority can never seem to reach their health goals.

Research has found that sleep deprivation has the same effect on your health as physical stress or illness. For example, when you're deprived of adequate sleep, hormones such as ghrelin (which signals hunger) and leptin (which signals satiety) can become imbalanced, leading to excessive appetite that can lead to a prediabetic state, inability to lose weight, increased blood pressure and premature aging.

When you're sleep deprived, your body also misses out on an important cleansing of the brain. While you are sleeping, your brain literally detoxes toxic waste and clears out your neurological cache via the glymphatic system. This system is similar to the lymphatic system, but the brain's glial cells manage it, hence the name "glymphatic." This cleansing system is ten times more active while you are sleeping, when your brain cells actually shrink about 60 percent, creating space for cerebrospinal fluid to flush out debris. This system is essential to eliminate harmful proteins potentially linked to such diseases as Alzheimer's.

So how much sleep is enough? Governments and many health experts have varying opinions on this. My advice is to find your own "sweet spot" for sleep. Generally speaking, for a healthy adult, adequate sleep is anywhere from seven and a half to nine hours a night. In the winter, when the days are shorter, your body naturally needs more sleep, whereas in the summer you may feel well rested after seven hours. **The key is to listen to your body.**

It's more difficult to achieve a natural, healthy glow when you are exhausted. There's a reason why it is called "beauty sleep."

Here are five strategies for a better sleep:

1. **Make sure the temperature of your bedroom does not exceed 68°F (20°C).** When you sleep, your body's temperature drops to its lowest level of the day. Keeping your bedroom too warm—above 75°F (24°C)—or too cool—below 54°F (12°C)—will interfere with your sleep because your body will constantly be trying to regulate its temperature.

2. **Sleep in complete darkness.** Melatonin and serotonin are hormones essential for a good night's sleep. There is a gland in your brain called the pineal gland, and when it senses light it will halt the release of these essential sleep hormones. Even the smallest sliver of light can disrupt sleep. I benefited tremendously when we got blackout curtains for our bedroom.

3. **Avoid artificial light from mobile devices, tablets and computers at least one and a half hours before sleep.** You've probably experienced this at some point—you feel tired but turn on your tablet only to feel totally awake two hours later. These devices emit a blue light that tricks the brain into thinking it's daytime and preventing the release of sleep hormones. Make sure you do not have any of these devices in your bedroom. If you must use your mobile device as your alarm clock, be sure to set it to airplane mode so it's not signalling back and forth with the cellphone tower all night—these waves can also be disruptive to your sleep.

4. **Take a warm bath before bed.** This habit is especially helpful if you've had a stressful day. When stress hormones are pumping, it is next to impossible to get into a calm, relaxed state and fall asleep. A warm bath with a relaxing essential oil like lavender (or a detox bath, as discussed on page 48) is the perfect habit just before bed to induce a restful sleep.

5. **Do a brain dump.** This is a wonderful habit I talked about in my first book, *Joyous Health*. Before bed, take out a piece of paper or a journal and write down everything on your mind without lifting your pen from the paper. Aim to fill an entire page with a constant stream of consciousness. This technique is also fantastic for emotional detoxification! If you've got a monkey brain that starts thinking about your to-do list as soon as you hit the sack, be sure to write it all down before you fall asleep.

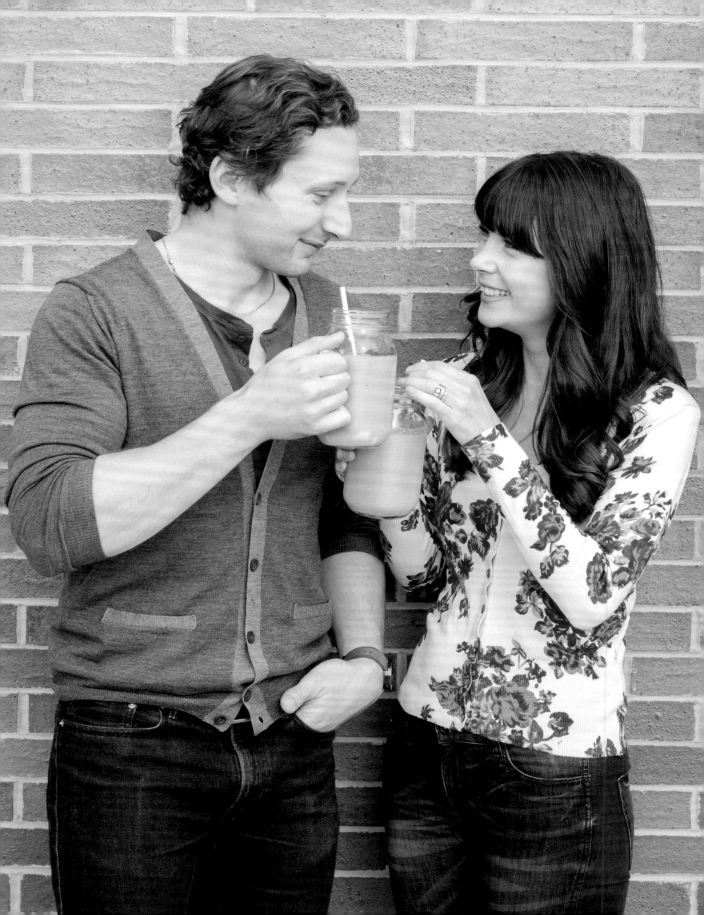

SOCIAL DETOX

My final point is something I always mention to clients and at public workshops: the importance of surrounding yourself with nourishing friends and family is just as essential as nourishing food. There's no end to the amount of research that shows that strong social ties and a sense of belonging truly enhance the quality of your life.

You don't need to be as severe as eliminating people from your life the way you might detox a food—it's much more passive than that. Simply take some time to evaluate all your relationships and make a priority of those who inspire and challenge you, whom you admire and vice versa. You will find that this simple detox habit dramatically improves your health and happiness.

Now that you know all the detox lifestyle habits available to you, choose the ones that really resonate with you the most. Rest assured you don't have to do all of these all at once. Focusing on just one new lifestyle habit each week will give you confidence to continue on this incredible and healing journey to feeling your most vibrant self.

Joyous Affirmation

Today is a wonderful opportunity to start fresh.
I am getting healthier and more vibrant
with each passing day.

4

SETTING UP YOUR JOYOUS DETOX-FRIENDLY KITCHEN

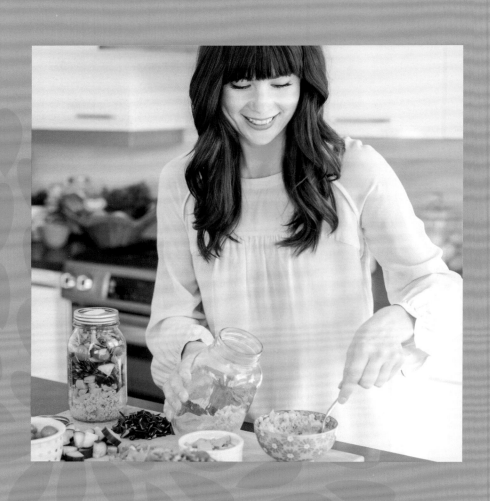

Your Joyous Detox starts in the kitchen. In this chapter, you will learn helpful tips to make over your kitchen. You'll get a "healthy swaps" chart, a list of essential kitchen equipment (plus some nice-to-haves), a list of healthy and detox-friendly foods to stock in your kitchen, and a few other handy charts, such as egg substitutions.

By the end of this chapter you'll be feeling very prepared—and excited!—to begin the Joyous Detox.

JOYOUS TIPS FOR A DETOX-FRIENDLY KITCHEN

1. Have a snack shelf in your fridge

The key to success is being prepared. Create a shelf in your fridge devoted to grab-and-go snacks so you are not tempted to eat junk when you're hungry. Here are some ideas for that snack shelf:

- **Cut-up veggie sticks.** The crunchier the better. When you chew something with a crunch, your brain acknowledges that you are actually eating. Enjoy veggies sticks with Creamy Cashew Veggie Dip (page 193) or Sunny Punchy Seed Spread (page 198).
- **Homemade trail mix.** Keeping it in the fridge keeps it fresher longer.
- **Fresh fruit.** Mix it up every week. Don't always buy the same fruit.
- **Roasted whole chicken.** Peel off chunks for a quick snack.
- **Coconut yogurt.** Enjoy with fresh fruit and chia seeds.
- **Joy's Favourite Breakfast Cookies** (page 115) or **No-Bake Superfood Breakfast Bars** (page 119).
- **Homemade chia jams** (pages 178–179).
- **Homemade dips and spreads** for crackers and vegetables (pages 193–198).
- **Nuts, seeds and nut butters** such as Cinnamon Pecan Butter (page 174). Always keep these in the fridge to prevent the good fats from going rancid.
- **Check out the recipes in "Salads and Snacks"** (page 170) for more ideas.

Keep non-perishables such as healthy crackers, dried fruit and other superfoods that don't need to be refrigerated on an easily accessible shelf in a kitchen cabinet.

If you have children, why not get them to spend some time with you in the kitchen helping to make some of these healthy snacks? Not only is it a great way for them to connect with real food, but when they come home from school and open the fridge they won't be saying, "There's nothing to eat!" because there will be plenty of healthy snacks on hand that they helped prepare.

2. Grocery shop at the same time each week

Let's face it, we are all busy—our careers and social lives are often the excuses we use when we don't make our health a priority. This is why scheduling time in your calendar for grocery shopping each week will establish a healthy routine. This will ensure you have a well-stocked kitchen, which is key to your success. If your kitchen is packed with healthy and yummy foods, then you'll be far less likely to eat junk.

3. Make a grocery list

This might sound pretty obvious, but how often do you actually write a list of what you need from the grocery store? When people don't write a list, they often end up spending more money and buying on impulse things that either are not healthy or they just don't need.

Did you know that North Americans waste 40 percent of their food each week because it rots in their fridge? What a waste of money! Decide before you shop what your meals are going to be for the week, then make a list of what you need for those meals. And once you're in the store, stick to that list. You'll reduce waste *and* save money! You can also keep a list handy in your kitchen and write down the basic items you're running low on throughout the week.

And remember, don't shop when you're hungry. You'll be tempted to buy junk foods!

4. Get rid of junk foods (but not by eating them)

As the old saying goes, "Out of sight, out of mind." Give your kitchen a makeover before beginning the detox. The same goes for your personal workspace and your car—remove temptation wherever it might be. Remember that the Joyous Detox is not meant to be for a limited time period. My hope is that while you're detoxing you love how you feel so much that it becomes a lifelong choice for you and your family. Therefore, there's simply no need for junk in your home!

5. Get rid of all those bottles of store-bought sauces and salad dressings

Get rid of foods with sneaky additives like excessive amounts of refined sugars. Refer back to chapter 1 for all the ingredients to avoid. You'll find that most store-bought sauces and salad dressings are full of chemicals and non-food substances. These are not detox friendly, despite any label telling you they're "low-fat" or "low-cal." Be sure to wash out and recycle all the bottles.

As you work your way through the recipes in this book, you'll discover that you'll never need another store-bought sauce or dressing again (with gluten-free tamari as the exception).

6. Get the right equipment

If your budget allows, make sure your kitchen is stocked with the right equipment (more on that in a bit) to make food prep as efficient as possible. I find that more often than not, people won't bat an eye at purchasing a new pair of shoes but wouldn't consider using that money for a spiralizer or blender instead. You'll have that piece of kitchen equipment far longer than any pair of shoes, and it will never go out of fashion!

7. Ditch the tin canned foods

In moderation, using canned foods that are BPA-free is okay. For example, when you need chickpeas in a pinch, using canned chickpeas is far more convenient than soaking and cooking them yourself. However, there should never be a need for canned fruits or vegetables. They often contain far too much sodium and, in the case of fruit, too much sugar. Furthermore, it is pretty gross when you think about the fact that the "best before date" can be years away, and it's chemicals that are preserving the food, not natural means of preserving such as fermenting or dehydrating. Fruits and vegetables should go bad!

8. Fresh is best and frozen comes second

If you shop once a week, you'll always have fresh on hand, but I recommend you have a few packages of frozen fruits or vegetables for convenience. Plus, frozen fruit in the months when fresh is out of season (think blueberries in the middle of January) is the best and most affordable option for making great smoothies. Frozen foods can actually be more nutrient-dense than fresh options, such as when certain fruits or vegetables are out of season. In winter, for example, frozen local strawberries are going to be far more nutrient-dense than fresh strawberries from New Zealand.

9. Choose safe pots and pans

Many non-stick pots and pans contain perfluorinated compounds, or PFCs, that are hazardous not only to the environment but also to humans. In fact, pet birds have been killed in seconds by chemicals emitting from a hot non-stick pan, in experiments done by the very same company that created these chemicals. The U.S. Environmental Protection Agency says PFCs "combine persistence, bio-accumulation, and toxicity properties to an extraordinary degree."

PFCs have been found in nearly all Americans tested by public health officials. These chemicals are associated with smaller birth weight and size in newborn babies, elevated cholesterol, abnormal thyroid hormones, liver inflammation and a weakened immune system, according to the Environmental Working Group.

Use cast-iron or stainless steel cookware instead or seek out non-stick pots and pans that are truly free of PFCs. If you're stuck with non-stick for now, then use it only at a very low temperature, never put it in the oven and make sure the exhaust fan is always on when you're cooking. As well, don't use the self-cleaning function on your oven, because there can be non-stick materials in your oven that contain—and emit—the same chemicals as your non-stick pans.

10. Choose safe food storage containers

Choose glass or stainless steel, or plastic containers labelled "BPA-free."

11. Use eco-friendly dish soap, dishwasher detergent and cleaning supplies

Cleaning supplies can contain hundreds of chemicals, and most of them are not safe. Have you ever thought about what that skull-and-crossbones image on your toilet bowl cleaner means? You get my point! Your local health store will have plenty of safe options for you that will help reduce your overall toxic load and are also better for the environment. Alternatively, you can find dozens of recipes for homemade dish soap, detergents and other cleaning supplies on the internet. As a bonus, you'll save some money too!

CLEAN OUT YOUR FRIDGE AND KITCHEN CABINETS

Take a couple of hours to go through your entire kitchen and give your food supply a bit of a makeover. Here is a healthy swaps chart to help you along, including recipe ideas to replace your unhealthy favourites with healthy and delicious new ones.

IS THIS IN YOUR KITCHEN?	STOCK THIS INSTEAD
BBQ sauce	Best Ever Homemade BBQ sauce (page 227)
Boxed cereal	Grain-Free Nutty Granola (page 114)
Canned fruits and vegetables	Fresh or flash-frozen
Canned soups	Fresh soup in glass jars, and homemade (pages 159–166)
Non-organic, plastic-bottled vegetable oils, including canola, soy, corn, safflower, sunflower	Organic coconut oil, grapeseed oil, extra-virgin olive oil, avocado oil, sesame oil, camelina oil. Choose oils in dark glass bottles.
Chocolate chips	Raw cacao nibs
Cocoa powder	Raw cacao powder
Condiments (sauces, spreads, etc.)	Spices, herbs, gluten-free tamari, garlic
Cow's milk	Nut milks: store-bought or homemade Nutty Milk (page 148)
Cow's milk cream	Coconut milk or coconut cream
Fruit juice	Fresh juices (pages 149–152)
Ice cream and other frozen treats	Freeze berries or grapes; to make your own frozen treats, just add ice to smoothies (pages 139–146)
Icing or frosting	Lemon Icing (page 256)
Jams	Chia jams (pages 178–179)
Ketchup	Avocado Tomato Salsa (page 203)
Margarine	Organic butter or coconut oil
Mayonnaise	Mashed avocado, Dijon mustard or Creamy Cashew Veggie Dip (page 193)
Milk chocolate	Dark chocolate
Milkshakes	Smoothies (pages 139–146)
Parmesan cheese	Nutritional yeast
Peanut butter	Cinnamon Pecan Butter (page 174); any other nut or seed butter
Pizza (takeout or frozen)	Portobello Mushroom Pizza Two Ways (page 234–235)
Prepared salad dressings	Homemade salad dressings (pages 183–201)
Pop	Kombucha or homemade drinks (pages 131–158)
Refined sugar	Stevia, honey, coconut sugar, applesauce, maple syrup
Salty snacks	Roasted chickpeas (pages 171–173)
Soft cheese	Mashed avocado
Table salt	Sea salt or Himalayan salt
White or whole wheat bread	Best Ever Cinnamon Flaxseed Bread (page 127)
White or whole wheat pasta	Zucchini Noodles (page 239), spaghetti squash or buckwheat noodles
White or whole wheat tortillas	Lettuce or brown rice tortillas
White rice	Cauliflower Rice (page 215) or quinoa

Now that you're an expert on making your kitchen detox friendly, let's talk about equipment essentials that every home cook and food lover deserves. Think of your tools as the paintbrushes an artist uses to create beautiful works of art!

EQUIPMENT ESSENTIALS

Blender

Every kitchen, whether you're detoxing or not, needs a good-quality blender. This kitchen essential will allow you to make everything from smoothies to an abundance of puréed foods such as soups, nut butters, hummus and pestos. (You may find food processors do a better job at nut butters and pestos, but more on that below.)

The wide price range among blenders, from inexpensive to outrageous, is usually due to the wattage (amount of blending power) and extra bells and whistles, including stainless steel bases and digital settings instead of buttons. A higher-wattage blender will do a more efficient job at pulverizing, while I've seen cheaper and lower-wattage blenders that can barely chew up spinach. A good blender is a worthwhile investment because you will have it for years. However, that doesn't mean you need to spend more than a few hundred dollars.

Price range: $100 to $500+
Brands: Blendtec, Breville, Oster, Vitamix

Good-quality chef's knife

Any chef will tell you that having good knives is essential to cooking with ease—and not cutting your fingers! However, it's not necessary to have an entire twenty-piece knife set if you want to save some dollars. Having one really good-quality chef's knife will allow you to do all the chopping and slicing you need to.

Unless you're a professional chef, it's probably not necessary to spend hundreds of dollars on a single knife. In Canada, you can find high-quality brands at Winners and HomeSense for half the price. Remember to sharpen your chef's knife every couple of weeks if you use it often.

Price range: $45 to $300+
Brands: Wüsthof, Zwilling J.A. Henckels

Food processor

Just like my blender, I use my food processor almost every day. Mini (2-cup/ 500 mL) food processors are fairly inexpensive and will do all the jobs a blender cannot do. I prefer my full-size food processor for nut butters, raw cookies and pestos because the blade is much larger and food particles never get stuck beneath the blade. If you have the budget, purchase a food processor that has two bowl sizes.

Price range: $50 to $500+, depending on whether you purchase
a mini food processor or one that has more than one bowl size
Brands: Breville, Cuisinart, KitchenAid

Wood cutting board

You'll be doing a lot of chopping during the Joyous Detox because what you'll be eating is predominantly plant-based, which means there are lots of vegetables to cut. A wood cutting board won't dull your knives like plastic, marble or glass do and keeps the knife from slipping so you have more control over what you're cutting.

You might be surprised to learn that, according to research from the University of California, Davis, plastic cutting boards harbour more bacteria than wood. Hardwoods pull down the bacteria and trap them deep inside, where they tend not to multiply and eventually die off, whereas bacteria remain on or close to the surface of plastic boards. Even when plastic cutting boards are put in the dishwasher, the bacteria just tend to spread around.

However, it is still important to keep your wood cutting board clean by washing it in hot water using an eco-friendly soap, especially if you have used it to cut any animal foods.

Good-quality cookware and bakeware

As mentioned earlier, avoid chemical non-stick coatings that contain PFCs. A number of non-stick brands are available that do not contain these chemicals. If you're not sure whether a pan is coated with these chemicals, contact the manufacturer. Older pots and pans will often be made of aluminum, which is also best avoided because exposure to aluminum may have negative effects on the nervous system.

There are many fantastic and affordable brands of stainless steel, copper and ceramic cookware; you'll just need to use a little extra coconut oil because they are generally not non-stick. A cast-iron grill pan can also be a handy piece of cookware for grilling chicken and fish. For baking root vegetables, I love my Le Creuset pots. They are super handy because you can use them on the stovetop and then transfer them to the oven.

I have a smorgasbord of different brands of cookware and bakeware. I suggest you do your research because each brand has its pros and cons, and some lines will have both eco-friendly and toxic cookware.

Brands: All-Clad, Calphalon, Ecolution, Le Creuset, Pyrex

Here are some small but very useful kitchen essentials:

- measuring cups and spoons
- vegetable peeler
- grater
- citrus juicer
- spatula
- large wooden spoons

Avoid plastic when you can. For example, measuring cups and spoons can be purchased in stainless steel or ceramic.

NICE-TO-HAVES

Juicer

There are two kinds of juicers on the market: slow juicers and centrifugal juicers. Slow juicers are the most effective, because they extract more juice from fruits and vegetables than a centrifugal juicer. They work by crushing and then pressing the fruits and vegetables to yield the most juice.

Centrifugal juicers extract juice by rapidly spinning the fruit or vegetable pulp, but the heat generated by this friction destroys many of the beneficial enzymes in the juice. However, centrifugal juicers do tend to be cheaper and they are faster.

In the slow juicer category, there are many different brands with varying settings and functions. Some slow juicers even make nut milk. The best thing to do when selecting a juicer is to read online reviews.

If you don't have the budget for a juicer, you can use your blender for any of the juice recipes in this book and strain out the pulp with a mesh strainer or a nut milk bag.

Price range: $150 to $500+
Brands: Breville, Hurom, Omega

Spiralizer

In the summer months, when there is an abundance of zucchini, I use my spiralizer at least once a week. It "spirals" vegetables into a noodle-like shape, hence the name. However, you can use a vegetable peeler and make flat, wide noodles instead.

Price range: $15 to $45

Indoor electric grill

This is a great tool if you don't have an outdoor grill. I use my indoor grill all year round for grilling everything from chicken to fish to tempeh. It is especially useful if you don't want to turn on the oven to grill something. Just be sure to investigate what kind of non-stick surface is used on the product you purchase.

A cast-iron grill pan for the stovetop is another great option and can be cheaper.

Price range: $60 to $450
Brands: All-Clad, Breville, Cuisinart, Hamilton Beach

Stand mixer

This is definitely a nice-to-have, but they're expensive. Even if a recipe doesn't call for an electric mixer, it can be helpful when you're mixing up muffin batter. I've had my stand mixer for over ten years. This is an appliance you will likely only ever need to purchase once.

Price range: $500+
Brands: Cuisinart, KitchenAid, Oster, Sunbeam

Rice cooker

A good friend of mine swears by his rice cooker for cooking everything from lentils to quinoa and, of course, rice. The best part of a rice cooker is that you just set the timer and walk away. When you're cooking quinoa or rice on the stovetop, you have to give it a stir every once in a while and keep an eye on it.

Price range: $35 to $100+
Brands: Aroma, Black & Decker, Hamilton Beach

Once you've cleaned out all the junk food from your kitchen, stocking it with delicious and nourishing foods will set the stage for a long, healthy life. Your kitchen is your personal pharmacy! As Hippocrates said, "Let food be thy medicine and medicine be thy food."

As I said earlier, rather than thinking of stocking your kitchen for the Joyous Detox as a short-term endeavour, think of this as a lifestyle change. Once you've given your kitchen a healthy makeover and stocked it with incredibly healing foods, you'll be well on your way to a healthy lifestyle for good. I encourage you to continue stocking your kitchen this way.

Rest assured that you don't have to toss out every single ingredient you have and completely restock your kitchen in order to follow the Joyous Detox. Just purchase what you need for the recipes you choose to make that week and try new recipes each week. This will help you build a Joyous Detox kitchen with each trip to the grocery store. This is a more budget-friendly and less overwhelming approach. It can take months to have a kitchen stocked with all these whole-food ingredients, but once you've begun to make these changes, your body will thank you!

KITCHEN STAPLES AND HOW TO STORE THEM

Kitchen pantry staples (non-perishables)

Fats and oils: coconut oil, coconut butter, extra-virgin olive oil, grapeseed oil, sesame oil, camelina oil

Flours: buckwheat flour, coconut flour, almond flour, brown rice flour

Grains and pseudograins: millet, short- and long-grain brown rice, black rice, quinoa, oats

Dried goods: beans, lentils, fruit, gluten-free pasta

Baking essentials: gluten-free and aluminum-free baking powder and baking soda, gluten-free chocolate chips, protein powder, dried fruit, coconut palm sugar, honey, coconut flakes

Herbs and spices: Keep a variety of dried herbs and spices, such as mixed Italian herbs, cardamom, cayenne, curry powder, garlic, turmeric, cinnamon, nutmeg and pepper. Choose organic as often as possible.

Condiments: sea salt or Himalayan rock salt, nutritional yeast, honey, balsamic vinegar, blackstrap molasses

Superfoods: raw cacao powder and nibs, protein powder, tea (various kinds), greens powder (once opened, be sure to refrigerate)

Jarred and canned foods: tomatoes, tomato paste, olives, unsweetened applesauce, organic BPA-free beans and lentils, organic BPA-free coconut milk, wild salmon in oil with the bones in

Joyous Tip

• • •

Once you've opened the package and exposed flour to the air, it's best to store it in an airtight container in the fridge or freezer to maintain freshness and prevent the naturally occurring oils in the flour from going rancid.

Refrigerated kitchen staples

Nut and seed butters: If you've not made them yourself, read your labels to make sure there are no sneaky and unnecessary ingredients added, such as oil, salt or sugar. These butters should have one ingredient: nuts or seeds.

Whole nuts and seeds: Stock your fridge with unsalted, unroasted nuts and seeds. You can salt and roast them yourself, if you like. You may wish to soak your nuts and seeds to increase their digestibility.

Nut milks: Avoid store-bought unless free of preservatives and additives. Generally speaking, the nut and seed milks that are found in the refrigerated section of the grocery store have fewer additives. That said, once you make your own nut milk, you'll never go back to store-bought again! Check out my Nutty Milk on page 148.

Whole eggs: preferably organic or "farm-fresh" from a local farmer who you know has good farming practices

Variety of fruits and vegetables: especially the "detox superfoods" listed in chapter 2

Fresh herbs: Keep a little herb garden on a windowsill. The most versatile herbs for cooking are basil, mint, oregano and cilantro. They can take any dish from mediocre to fabulous.

Fermented foods: kimchi, miso, sauerkraut, apple cider vinegar, gluten-free tamari (if you are soy-sensitive, "coconut-aminos" are a great alternative to tamari)

Condiments: Dijon mustard, maple syrup, hot sauce

Other: ghee, organic butter

Joyous Tip

• • •

Fresh is best, but it's not always possible. Even though canned foods are convenient, limit your consumption of them. Try to keep them for emergencies or as a last resort, such as using canned tomatoes in the winter.

• • •

Variety is key! Every week your fresh produce will probably look a little different and will definitely vary from month to month, depending on what is in season and available. Remember, it is important to avoid getting stuck in a rut eating the same foods week after week. Be sure to check out the meal plans in the next chapter for inspiration.

Frozen kitchen staples

Protein: fish, chicken, turkey

Frozen fruits and vegetables: Variety is key, just like with fresh fruits and vegetables. Keeping frozen produce on hand is great for last-minute meals and wonderful for smoothies. Make sure you give the bag of frozen produce a good feel to ensure it is not suffering from freezer burn.

Joyous Tip

• • •

When you purchase fish that is not frozen, be sure to ask if it has been "previously frozen." If it has, you should not freeze it again. You should only freeze truly *fresh* fish. If you thaw previously frozen fish a second time it is more likely to harbour bacteria.

For sustainable fish and seafood choices, look for varieties certified by Ocean Wise.

SHOULD YOU PURCHASE ORGANIC?

Every year, the Environmental Working Group updates their "Dirty Dozen," which lists the fruits and vegetables with the highest levels of pesticides, and their "Clean Fifteen," which are the fruits and vegetables with the lowest levels of pesticides. To reduce unnecessary exposure to pesticides, buy organic varieties of the "Dirty Dozen" foods as often as possible.

WHERE TO SHOP?

Most major grocery stores now have a natural foods section where you will be able to find staples such as coconut flour, nut butters, fresh and frozen organic produce and more. Local health food stores and farmers' markets are my favourite places to shop for healthy food.

If the grocery store closest to you does not have a wide variety of health foods, I suggest shopping online. You can find great options for both non-perishable foods and natural personal care products. For fresh produce, consider an organic delivery service or CSA box.

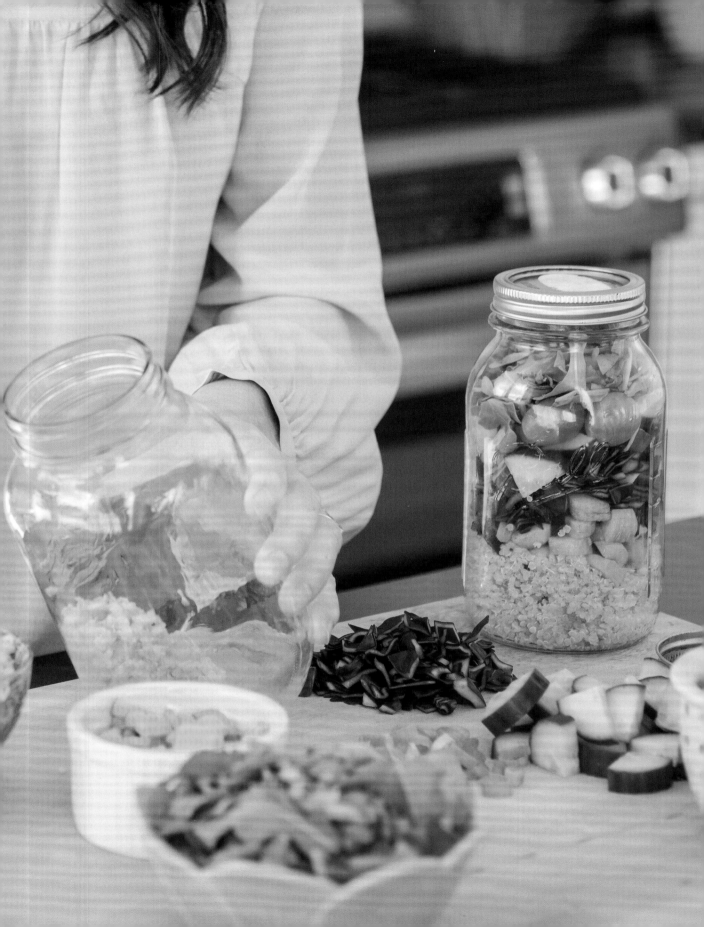

COOKING TEMPERATURES FOR FATS AND OILS

Oils begin to break down at a certain temperature known as their "smoke point." When heated past their smoke point, oils release free radicals, which aren't healthy for you. Overheated oils can form other harmful compounds such as lipid peroxides and aldehydes, which may contribute to cancer.

Generally speaking, the more saturated fat an oil contains, the more stable during cooking it is. This chart provides you with guidance on temperatures for the oils I've used in my recipes.

Always choose organic, cold-pressed oils sold in dark glass bottles.

HEALTHY OILS AND THEIR USES		
OIL	BEST FOR	AVOID
Avocado oil	Baking; sautéing medium to high temperature	Frying
Camelina oil	Baking; sautéing medium to high temperature	Frying
Coconut oil*	Baking; sautéing medium temperature	Frying
Extra-virgin olive oil**	Salad dressings; drizzling on food after cooking and low- to medium-temperature cooking. You can always dilute it with a touch of water when sautéing with it.	High-temperature sautéing or frying
Flaxseed oil	Salad dressings; smoothies	All cooking methods. Must be kept refrigerated.
Grapeseed oil	Baking; sautéing medium to high temperature	Frying
Sesame oil	Salad dressings; drizzling on food after cooking; low- to medium-temperature cooking	High-temperature sautéing or frying

*   Choose unrefined coconut oil. Refined coconut oil might stand up to heat better and have no coconut taste, but it is, well, refined. Coconut oil should in fact smell and taste like coconut, so avoid coconut oil that has "deodorized" on the label.

** For years, extra-virgin olive oil has had a bad rap as a cooking oil, but research shows this might not be warranted. The quality of the oil really determines the smoke point, and there is a broad variation in quality from one brand to another. Unadulterated high-quality extra-virgin olive oil contains many antioxidants that protect the oil at high temperatures. Cheaper olive oils will smoke at a relatively low temperature. The lesson here is to buy the best-quality extra-virgin olive oil for the best nutrition, taste and safe smoke point.

EGG SUBSTITUTIONS

Even though eggs are a detox-friendly food, many people have allergies or sensitivities to them. Here is an easy chart to follow if you need to avoid eggs. (Please note that I have not tested my recipes with these substitutions.)

EGG SUBSTITUTIONS				
CHIA SEEDS	**GROUND FLAXSEEDS**	**COMBINATION OF GROUND AND/OR SPROUTED CHIA/FLAX**	**APPLESAUCE**	**BANANA**
1 tbsp (15 mL) chia seeds	1 tbsp (15 mL) ground flaxseeds	1 tbsp (15 mL) mixed chia/flax	¼ cup (60 mL) unsweetened applesauce	½ medium ripe banana
+ ¼ cup (60 mL) water	+ 3 tbsp (45 mL) water	+ ¼ cup (60 mL) water		
= 1 egg	= 1 egg	= 1 egg	= 1 egg	= 1 egg
Let sit for 10 minutes	Let sit for 10 minutes	Let sit for 10 minutes		

Note: If a recipe calls for more than 2 eggs, these substitutions are less likely to be effective.

Joyous Affirmation

I have all the energy I need to accomplish my goals.

5

JOYOUS DETOX
MEAL PLANS

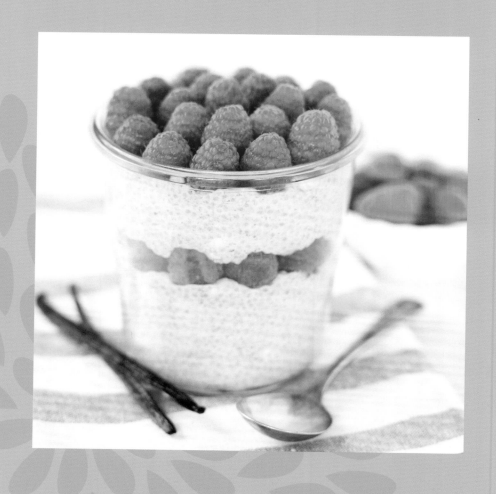

Congratulations! You've made it to the chapter with the Joyous Detox meal plans to help guide you joyously through your detoxification.

You'll find a nourishing 2-Day Reboot Detox meal plan and both omnivore and vegan/vegetarian 10-Day Joyous Detox meal plans to choose from, along with a 10-Day Joyous Lifestyle Detox.

Remember, this is *your* detox, so you may wish to skip the suggested meal plans altogether and just choose recipes from the book that appeal most to you. I think you will find they are all delicious, so you won't have any trouble choosing!

At the end of this chapter I've included a number of frequently asked questions to help guide you along.

I'm very excited for you to begin, because most people have no idea how good their body is designed to feel until they take a break from certain foods and enjoy super-nourishing detox-friendly recipes like the ones in these meal plans. When you make eating this way part of your everyday life, as opposed to doing it only for a short time, it will put you on the path to joyous health for life.

PRE-CLEANSING

If you are not already eating detox-friendly foods and living a detox lifestyle, I highly recommend you do a pre-cleanse. Pre-cleansing simply helps ease your body into the Joyous Detox and lessens any negative side effects that you might encounter. If you've been eating the Standard American Diet for the past several years, or even decades, then pre-cleansing will make the detox changes less of a shock to your system.

I suggest you pre-cleanse for at least seven days before the Joyous Detox.

Here are simple guidelines to follow for a successful pre-cleanse:

- Each morning, on an empty stomach, drink a large glass of filtered water with freshly squeezed lemon juice in it. If you are concerned about the enamel on your teeth, swish plain water around your mouth afterwards.
- Slowly cut back on coffee consumption so that by the time you're ready to detox you are no longer drinking coffee. See page 96 for a coffee detox.
- Increase your water consumption, if necessary. Your urine should be pale yellow. This may mean drinking 8 cups (2 L) of water a day. You may need to drink even more, depending on your level of activity and the climate where you live.
- Eliminate all forms of junk and fast food. Refer to the list of what to ditch on page 3, especially when it comes to food additives. Start reading the labels on any packaged food you buy.
- Cook your own food as often as possible.
- Choose a detox superfood to enjoy at every meal and snack. Refer to chapter 2 for a list of superfoods.

- Choose organic more often. Buying organic whenever possible means you'll avoid a lot of toxic pesticides. If you're worried about the cost of buying exclusively organic, consider buying just the "Dirty Dozen" in the organics section.
- You may want to enjoy a smoothie each morning for breakfast for the duration of the pre-cleanse. See pages 139–146 for recipes.

Once you've done this for seven days, you're ready for the Joyous Detox!

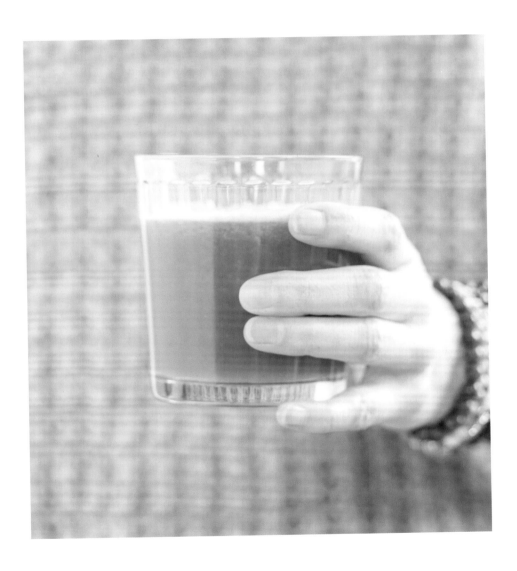

2-DAY REBOOT DETOX

This detox is called a "reboot" because it's ideal for those times when maybe you've overindulged a little and need to hit the reset button. This will give you the confidence to get back on track with your health goals. Sometimes we just need a little reminder that we are totally capable of steering ourselves in the right direction—toward incredible health and vitality.

Choose two days when you do not have any social obligations and you can concentrate on having a stress-free experience. A weekend would be a great time to do this 2-Day Reboot Detox.

You may find that you have plenty of leftovers to enjoy after the two days are complete.

Note: You can do this Reboot Detox at any time. It does not have to be preceded by a pre-cleanse.

TWO-DAY REBOOT DETOX MEAL PLAN		
MEAL	**DAY 1**	**DAY 2**
BEFORE BREAKFAST	Freshly squeezed lemon and water or Beet and Strawberry Detox Juice (page 151)	Freshly squeezed lemon and water or Green Sparkle Juice (page 152)
BREAKFAST	Green Sparkle Smoothie (page 139)	Joyous Energy Smoothie (page 141)
MID-MORNING SNACK	Chia Seed Blueberry Drink (page 133)	Chia Seed Blueberry Drink (page 133)
LUNCH	Any mason jar salad (pages 188–191) + Creamy Cashew Veggie Dip (page 193) with cut-up vegetables	Superfood Salad with Creamy Dressing (page 201) + Creamy Cashew Veggie Dip (page 193) with cut-up vegetables
MID-AFTERNOON SNACK	Detox Ginger Tea (page 131) + Chocolate Chia Mousse (page 252)	Detox Ginger Tea (page 131) + 2 Energy Booster Balls (page 181)
DINNER	Mint Guacamole Lettuce Wraps (page 220) + Purple and Green Cabbage Slaw (page 233)	Sesame Orange Quinoa Bowl (page 230)

10-DAY JOYOUS DETOX

The first meal plan I've given you is the ideal 10-day detox if you eat animal foods such as eggs and fish. Protein is extremely helpful for liver detoxification because amino acids, which are derived from protein, help to make the enzymes involved in detoxification processes.

If you're a vegan or vegetarian, you'll find a suitable 10-day detox meal plan follows the omnivore version.

Even though these are detox-friendly meals, I'm quite certain you will not feel deprived. Focus on how well you are treating your body and give yourself a pat on the back because you are doing something amazing for yourself!

If you are doing this detox on your own and follow the meal plan exactly, you may find that you have plenty of leftovers each day. I would suggest you freeze the leftovers to enjoy after the detox.

A NOTE ON SNACKING

In all my detox plans, the snacking ideas are just suggestions. You may find that some days you are hungrier than others, so the snacks may come in handy to tide you over until the next meal. On other days, you may sail through the day without wanting any snacks. Every person and every day is different, so the key is to *listen to your body*. You may find you need a mid-morning *and* a mid-afternoon snack, and that is okay! Nevertheless, try to avoid going longer than four hours without eating.

Joyous Tip

• • •

What about dessert? Desserts are meant to be an occasional treat, which is why they are not listed in the meal plans. Use your discretion about when to include a dessert. You may wish to consider avoiding all forms of natural sugars for the entire 10 days—or not. It's up to you! Some of my favourite dessert recipes in this book are the Raspberry Vanilla Bean Chia Pudding (page 259), Chocolate Chia Mousse (page 252) and Baked Brown Rice Pudding (page 250).

10-DAY JOYOUS DETOX OMNIVORE MEAL PLAN

MEAL	DAY 1	DAY 2	DAY 3	DAY 4	DAY 5	
BEFORE BREAKFAST	Freshly squeezed lemon and water or Refreshing Green Juice (page 149)	Freshly squeezed lemon and water or Beet and Strawberry Detox Juice (page 151)	Freshly squeezed lemon and water or Basil Lime Juice (page 152)	Freshly squeezed lemon and water or Green Sparkle Juice (page 152)	Freshly squeezed lemon and water or Beet and Strawberry Detox Juice (page 151)	
BREAKFAST	Coconut Yogurt Parfait with Chia Jam (page 110)	Rejuvenate Me Smoothie (page 146)	Joy's Favourite Breakfast Cookie (page 115) + Green Sparkle Juice (page 152)	Superfood Quinoa Bowl (page 124)	Blueberry Bliss Smoothie Bowl (page 147)	
LUNCH	Superfood Salad with Creamy Dressing (page 201)	Leftover chilled Salmon Quinoa Cake (page 229) + Purple and Green Cabbage Slaw (page 233)	Mint Guacamole Lettuce Wraps (page 220)	Any mason jar salad (pages 188–191)	Citrus Fennel Salad with Toasted Sunflower Seeds (page 184) + Hummus with cut-up vegetables	
DINNER	Salmon Quinoa Cakes with Lemon Sauce (page 229) + Mixed leafy green salad	Zucchini Noodles with Avocado Cream Sauce (page 239)	Chicken Quinoa Stew (page 162)	Fish "Tacos" with Mango Avocado Salsa (page 223) + Cucumber Watermelon Salad (page 202)	Juicy Chicken Spinach Burgers (page 224) + Everything but the Kitchen Sink Salad with Creamy Dijon Dressing (page 192)	
SNACKS	Sea Salt Rosemary Roasted Chickpeas (page 173)	Energy Booster Balls (page 181) (freeze extras)	Any chia seed drink (pages 133–134)	Energy Booster Balls (page 181)	Best Ever Cinnamon Flaxseed Bread (page 127) with any chia jam (pages 178–179)	

MEAL	DAY 6	DAY 7	DAY 8	DAY 9	DAY 10
BEFORE BREAKFAST	Freshly squeezed lemon and water or Refreshing Green Juice (page 149)	Freshly squeezed lemon and water or Green Sparkle Juice (page 152)	Freshly squeezed lemon and water or Beet and Strawberry Detox Juice (page 151)	Freshly squeezed lemon and water or Basil Lime Juice (page 152)	Freshly squeezed lemon and water or Refreshing Green Juice (page 149)
BREAKFAST	Buckwheat Pancakes with Warmed Blueberries (page 105)	No-Bake Superfood Breakfast Bar (page 119)	Blueberry Bliss Smoothie Bowl (page 147)	Green Sparkle Smoothie (page 139)	No-Bake Superfood Breakfast Bar (page 119)
LUNCH	Refreshing Sweet Pea Soup (page 166)	Soothing Golden Smoothie (page 144) + Creamy Cashew Veggie Dip (page 193) with cut-up vegetables	Chickpea Burgers (page 216) + Everything but the Kitchen Sink Salad with Creamy Dijon Dressing (page 192)	Any mason jar salad (pages 188–191) + Energy Booster Ball (page 181)	Guacamole Devilled Eggs (page 120) + Creamy Cashew Veggie Dip (page 193) with cut-up veggies
DINNER	Any portobello mushroom pizza (page 234–235) + Mixed greens with Best Ever Hemp Caesar Salad Dressing (page 199)	Walker's Chicken with Fennel, Orange and Mint (page 240)	Spicy Cacao Chicken Tortillas (page 219)	Fish "Tacos" with Mango Avocado Salsa (page 223)	Black Rice Butternut Squash Salad (page 187)
SNACKS	Cinnamon Pecan Butter (page 174) with sliced apple	Sunny Punchy Seed Spread (page 198) with cucumber slices	Blueberry Chia Jam (page 178) on gluten-free crackers	Cinnamon Roasted Chickpeas (page 171)	Apple Pie Bites (page 260)

10-DAY JOYOUS DETOX VEGAN MEAL PLAN (WITH VEGETARIAN OPTIONS)

MEAL	DAY 1	DAY 2	DAY 3	DAY 4	DAY 5
BEFORE BREAKFAST	Freshly squeezed lemon and water or Green Sparkle Juice (page 152)	Freshly squeezed lemon and water or Beet and Strawberry Detox Juice (page 151)	Freshly squeezed lemon and water or Basil Lime Juice (page 152)	Freshly squeezed lemon and water or Refreshing Green Juice (page 149)	Freshly squeezed lemon and water or Beet and Strawberry Detox Juice (page 151)
BREAKFAST	Coconut Yogurt Parfait with Chia Jam (page 110) *Vegetarian option:* Family Veggie Frittata (page 109)	Rejuvenate Me Smoothie (page 146) *Vegetarian option:* Joy's Favourite Breakfast Cookie (page 115)	No-Bake Superfood Breakfast Bar (page 119) *Vegetarian option:* Cinnamon Toast with Pecan Butter and Chia Jam (page 123)	Superfood Quinoa Bowl (page 124)	Strawberry Oat Mini Pancakes (page 103) *Vegetarian option:* Guacamole Devilled Eggs (page 120)
LUNCH	Superfood Salad with Creamy Dressing (page 201)	Purple and Green Cabbage Slaw (page 204) + Gluten-free crackers with Avocado Tomato Salsa (page 203)	Mint Guacamole Lettuce Wraps (page 220)	Any mason jar salad (pages 188–191)	Citrus Fennel Salad with Toasted Sunflower Seeds (page 184) + Sun-Dried Tomato Olive Spread (page 196) with gluten-free crackers
DINNER	Grilled Tempeh Kebabs with the Best Ever Homemade BBQ Sauce (page 227) + Mixed leafy green salad	Zucchini Noodles with Avocado Cream Sauce (page 239)	Black Rice Butternut Squash Salad (page 187)	Warm Sweet Potato Kale Bowl with Quinoa (page 213) *Vegetarian option:* Chickpea Burger (page 216) + Sun-Dried Tomato Olive Spread (page 196) with gluten-free crackers or chopped crunchy vegetables	Everything but the Kitchen Sink Salad with Creamy Dijon Dressing (page 192) + Chickpea Blender Soup (page 161)
SNACKS	Energy Booster Balls (page 181)	Creamy Cashew Veggie Dip (page 193) with cut-up vegetables	Any chia seed drink (pages 133–134)	Energy Booster Balls (page 181)	Cinnamon Pecan Butter (page 174) with sliced apple

MEAL	DAY 6	DAY 7	DAY 8	DAY 9	DAY 10
BEFORE BREAKFAST	Freshly squeezed lemon and water or Refreshing Green Juice (page 149)	Freshly squeezed lemon and water or Green Sparkle Juice (page 152)	Freshly squeezed lemon and water or Basil Lime Juice (page 152)	Freshly squeezed lemon and water or Refreshing Green Juice (page 149)	Freshly squeezed lemon and water or Basil Lime Juice (page 152)
BREAKFAST	Matcha Green Tea Smoothie (page 145)	Grain-Free Nutty Granola (page 114) with coconut yogurt	Overnight Oatmeal with Peaches and Apricots (page 123)	No-Bake Superfood Breakfast Bar (page 119) *Vegetarian option:* Family Veggie Frittata (page 109)	Soothing Golden Smoothie (page 144) *Vegetarian option:* Joy's Favourite Breakfast Cookie (page 115) + Green Sparkle Juice (page 152)
LUNCH	Purple Cabbage Walnut Meat "Tacos" (page 233)	Soothing Golden Smoothie (page 144) + Creamy Cashew Veggie Dip (page 193) with cut-up vegetables *Vegetarian option:* Family Veggie Frittata (page 109)	Purple Cabbage Walnut Meat "Tacos" (page 233) *Vegetarian option:* Guacamole Devilled Eggs (page 120) + Superfood Salad with Creamy Dressing (page 201)	Sweet Potato Coconut Soup (page 159) + Everything but the Kitchen Sink Salad with Creamy Dijon Dressing (page 192)	Sweet Potato Coconut Soup (page 159) + Sun-Dried Tomato Olive Spread (page 196) with gluten-free crackers
DINNER	Portobello Mushroom Pizza (page 234) + Mixed greens with Best Ever Hemp Caesar Salad Dressing (page 199) sprinkled with Sea Salt Rosemary Roasted Chickpeas (page 173)	Sesame Orange Quinoa Bowl (page 230)	Warm Sweet Potato Kale Bowl with Quinoa (page 213)	Zucchini Noodles with Avocado Cream Sauce (page 239) *Vegetarian option:* Chickpea Burger (page 216) + Crunch-tastic Sauerkraut (page 205) + Roasted Balsamic Kale (page 226)	Sesame Orange Quinoa Bowl (page 230)
SNACKS	Chocolate Chia Mousse (page 252) *Vegetarian option:* Pumpkin Chocolate Chip Mini Muffin (page 245)	Cinnamon Roasted Chickpeas (page 171)	Hemp Heart Spinach Spread (page 182) with cucumber slices	Chia Seed Blueberry Drink (page 133)	Hemp Heart Spinach Spread (page 182) with cucumber slices

10-DAY LIFESTYLE DETOX

You can do this detox alongside one of the 10-day meal plans, or on its own at any time.

10-DAY LIFESTYLE DETOX		
DAY 1	Connect	Reach out to someone you really enjoy being around and make a date to spend some time with them in the very near future.
DAY 2	Detox Bath	Take a detox bath. See page 48 for a how-to.
DAY 3	Vitamin G	Spend at least 45 minutes in nature today. Greenspace (where the G comes in) is essential for recharging your personal battery and is proven to uplift your spirit and put you in a good mood.
DAY 4	Personal Care Detox	Take some time to review all your personal care products to ensure they do not contain the "Toxic Ten" listed on page 57. I've provided you with some strategies to avoid these chemicals on page 58.
DAY 5	Dry Skin Brushing	Purchase a dry skin brush and learn about this essential detox habit on page 49. I personally enjoy this detox habit every single day, but you can start out with at least three times a week. Dry skin brushes are available at most health food stores.
DAY 6	Digital Detox	It's likely been a while since you've disconnected from all forms of digital media. Take a deliberate break from your mobile device and computer today. Learn more about this on page 52.
DAY 7	Get a massage	Do something nice for yourself today and book a massage. I probably don't need to tell you how amazing you'll feel afterward. If you are on a budget, consider booking with a student at a massage therapy school.
DAY 8	Sweat it out	Book yourself a good sweat session in an infrared sauna.
DAY 9	Social Detox	Take some time to do a social detox. Learn more about this detox habit on page 63.
DAY 10	Meditation	Quiet your mind by taking five minutes for meditation today. For a quick how-to, see page 53.

FREQUENTLY ASKED QUESTIONS

Here I've compiled the questions I'm most frequently asked when I teach workshops on detoxing. These include how to detox from coffee, what to do if you're craving sugar and how to check your "transit time."

Please keep in mind that the Joyous Detox does not override any medical advice you receive. This detox is not meant to treat any illness or disease. If you have questions related to your health and this detox, speak with your medical professional.

Will I experience any unpleasant symptoms while detoxing?

It is possible that you may experience any of the following: fatigue, headache, flu-like symptoms, hunger, changes in digestion (constipation or diarrhea), bad breath, body odour, moodiness and skin breakouts. Usually, these symptoms do not last longer than one to three days. These symptoms will be more intense the poorer your diet and nutrition were before you began the Joyous Detox. Drinking more water and getting adequate rest is the best solution for most of these symptoms. If you continue to feel unwell, though, it's best to stop the detox.

These symptoms can occur for two reasons. First, removing junk from your diet may cause symptoms similar to those experienced with withdrawal from addictive substances such as drugs and alcohol. Second, eating foods that stimulate detoxification can make you temporarily feel ill if you are not effectively eliminating them. This is why I am not a fan of juice-only cleansing, because it awakens a lot of toxic matter. If you rate your health and digestion a 10 out of 10, meaning all your channels of elimination are finely tuned and effective at eliminating the toxic junk you are awakening from juicing, then juicing is safe, but most people do not fall into this category. If you do not have an effective digestive system and you are not eating any fibre because you are just juicing, you may start to feel very ill because you are not eliminating toxins effectively via your bowels.

Will my digestion be affected during the detox?

With any change in diet, digestion is almost always affected—in this case, positively. You may experience a short-term increase in gassiness or bloating if your body is not used to fibre, but you will quickly adjust. You'll likely find that if you normally suffer from bloating, it will drastically improve during the detox.

If you are not used to eating a lot of roughage, such as raw fruits and vegetables, and an increase in raw foods makes you feel more bloated, cut back on raw foods and choose more recipes that include cooked foods.

If you notice a dramatic improvement in your digestive system during the detox, you may want to further investigate possible food sensitivities and intolerances with a natural healthcare practitioner.

When should I start the Joyous Detox?

There will never be a perfect time to detox, but you generally want to do a detox when you can carve out time in your schedule to make healthy meal preparation a priority. Many people like to do a detox in January, after the December holidays, or after any other times of overindulgence, such as a week at the cottage. Spring is one of the best times for detoxing because nature is providing an abundance of detox-friendly foods. Many people do a spring clean of their home, so it is also a great time to do a spring clean of your body!

Can I do the detox if I am breastfeeding or pregnant?

The short answer is no to both. The longer answer is that if you already eat nourishing, healthy foods, there is no reason you cannot enjoy some of the delicious recipes found in this book. If you are pregnant, there may be an ingredient you might want to avoid, such as matcha. The best thing to do is show the recipes you want to try to your natural healthcare practitioner and get the okay from them so you feel confident with your choices. If you focus on whole, real food, there should be no issues. I ate recipes from this book while I was pregnant and while breastfeeding.

Is there any other time I shouldn't detox?

Generally speaking, if you are ill, recovering from illness, undergoing a medical treatment or going through a stressful situation, then it is best to avoid detoxing. If you feel unwell, it is better to determine and address the underlying cause of your condition and discuss it with your natural healthcare practitioner before beginning the detox.

If you are taking a course of antibiotics or undergoing chemotherapy or radiation, it would be best to postpone the detox until you are better. However, there are still many recipes in this book that you can enjoy.

Can I take my regular supplements during a detox?

Most likely, yes, especially if you take a multivitamin or probiotic. However, it's best to talk to your natural healthcare practitioner about which supplements you should continue and which you may want to take a break from. Be sure to let them know you are doing a whole-foods detox that is not assisted by herbs (unless you are drinking a detox-friendly tea every day). Show them the recipes in this book.

Can I have desserts?

You may have noticed that the 2-Day Reboot and 10-Day Detoxes do not include any desserts. It is up to you whether you have a dessert or not. You may wish to take a break from all forms of sugar, including natural sugars, for the duration of the detox. You can enjoy the recipes in the "Sweets and Treats" section (page 245) if you are embarking on this journey as a "detox lifestyle," not a time-restricted endeavour.

How do I detox from caffeine, specifically coffee?

I do not recommend you drink caffeinated beverages, such as coffee or pop, during the detox. Caffeine acts like a drug in the body, so when you suddenly remove the drug, your body will experience withdrawal symptoms such as caffeine-induced headaches. Here is how you can help reduce the symptoms of caffeine withdrawal leading up to the detox.

Coffee Detox—Based on two cups of coffee per day
Week 1: Cut back to one and a half cups of coffee a day.
Week 2: Cut back to one cup of coffee a day.
Week 3: Drink one Americano a day. (One shot of espresso contains only 75 mg of caffeine, while a mug of drip coffee can contain over 250 mg.)
Week 4: Cut out coffee completely and instead drink green tea, which has anywhere from 25 to 50 mg of caffeine per cup.

Dandy Blend is my favourite herbal coffee substitute. It smells, tastes and brews like instant coffee. Add some cinnamon and raw honey to it and it becomes a very tasty, comforting hot drink.

How do I check my "transit time"?

Your transit time is how long it takes for food to be digested and eliminated. This is valuable information because it can determine how sluggish or effective your digestive system is.

Here's what you do: Buy some raw beets, wash them and, if they are not organic, peel off the skin. Using a cheese grater or mandoline, grate the beets and mix them into a salad. It is best to eat them raw.

After you've eaten the beets, look in the toilet after each bowel movement and take note when you see a red colour in your stools. Do not be alarmed! This can be quite shocking the first time you see it. You may also notice your urine turns pinkish or red, a phenomenon called beeturia.

The optimal bowel transit time is 12 to 24 hours. If you don't see red until days later, you will definitely benefit from the Joyous Detox because a slow transit time or constipation is a surefire sign you need to detox. If you are concerned, speak with your natural healthcare practitioner.

How will I get calcium if I don't eat dairy?

There are plenty of plant-based foods that are good sources of calcium, including chives, radishes, seaweeds, leeks, potatoes, leafy greens (spinach, kale, arugula, watercress, beet greens), garlic, parsley, tahini, spirulina, nuts and seeds.

Can I exercise while detoxing?

It's really up to you. Listen to your body, because every person is unique. Take it easy during the detox. Ideally, walking, cycling, lifting light weights or yoga will be sufficient. I do not recommend starting a detox while training for a marathon or doing similar intense activity. If you do light activity and do not feel your best, take a break until you've finished detoxing. As I've mentioned many times throughout this book, my hope is that you continue eating this way long after the detox is finished. If at first you feel very lethargic or have any of the unpleasant symptoms mentioned earlier, you will probably find they ease up as the detox progresses.

I'm craving sugar. What should I do?

Cravings are usually short-lived and can result from not eating enough protein and fat or they may have an emotional cause. Keeping a wellness journal can help you determine the cause of your cravings. Are you craving cookies and ice cream after a stressful day at work? If so, find an outlet other than food, such as going for a walk, calling a friend or knitting. If the craving is more physiological in origin, make sure you are eating enough fat and protein. Craving chocolate ice cream? Make the Chocolate Chia Mousse on page 252 instead and you'll forget all about that ice cream craving.

I have an event to go to where I know there won't be detox-friendly options to eat. What should I do?

Stay committed to your detox. You can do it! Simply eat before going to the event and let people know you are doing a detox so you won't be pressured into drinking alcohol or eating junk foods. If it's a family event, make something from this book to bring.

Joyous Affirmation

I am joyful and excited as positive changes
enter my life. I am vibrant and alive!

6

JOYOUS DETOX
RECIPES

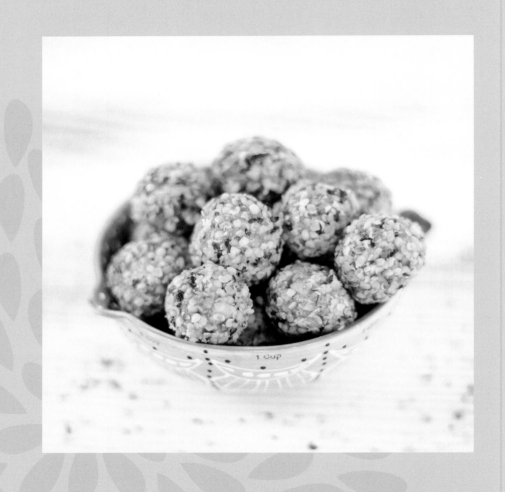

(GF) Gluten-free

(SF) Sugar-free

(V) Vegetarian
(may include eggs)

(RSF) Refined Sugar-free

(V) Vegan
(no animal products)

(DF) Dairy-free

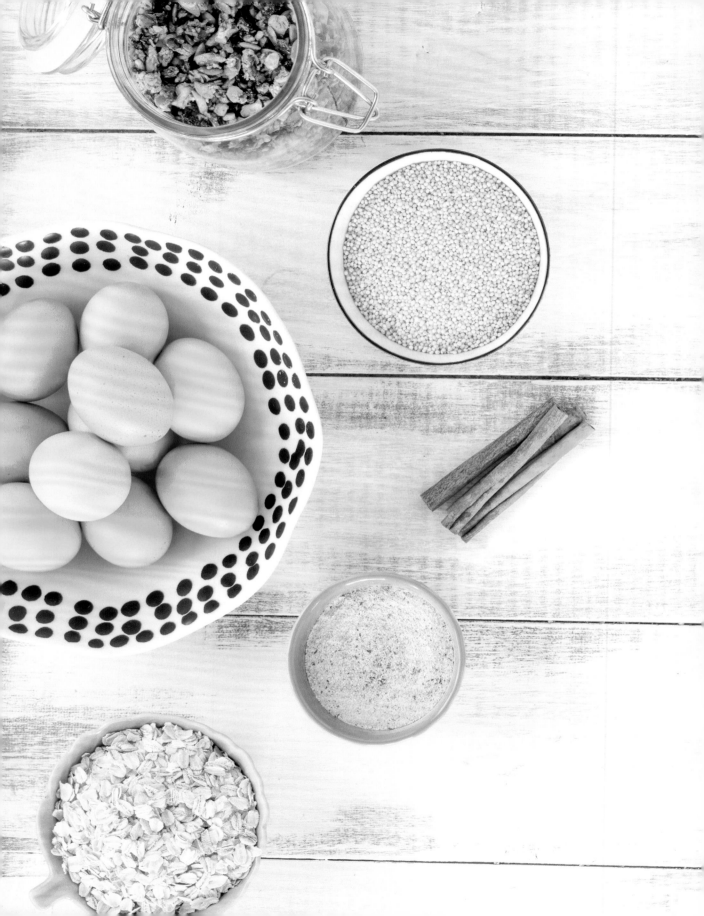

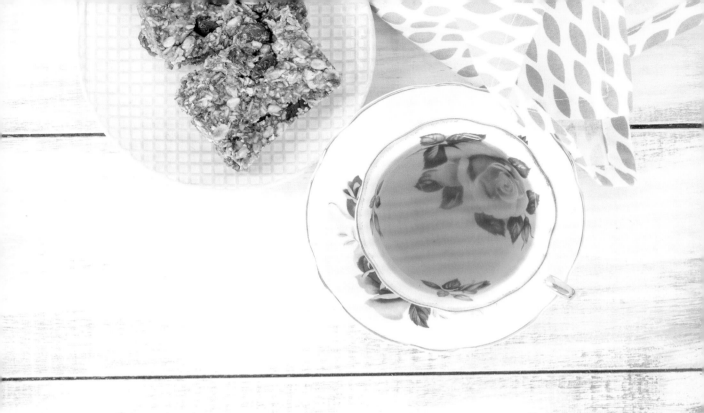

RISE and SHINE

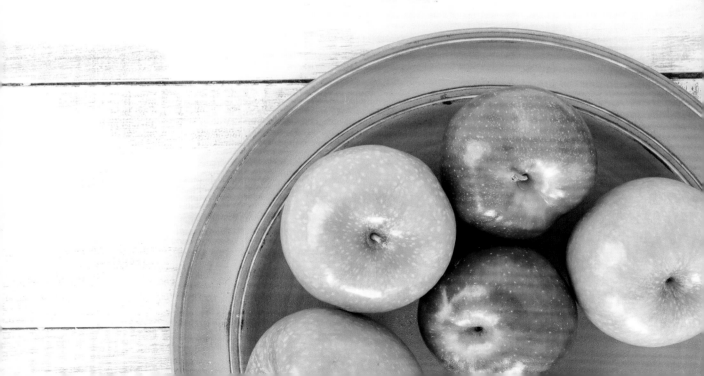

Strawberry Oat Mini Pancakes

These are my favourite "fast food" pancakes on weekday mornings. If I'm making them just for myself I freeze the leftovers and pop them in my toaster to enjoy another day.

Makes 10 mini pancakes

 Vegetarian   Gluten-free   Dairy-free   Refined Sugar-free

2 cups (500 mL) old-fashioned rolled oats*

1 cup (250 mL) filtered water

1 cup (250 mL) strawberries, finely chopped

1 banana, mashed

1 egg, whisked

½ tsp (2 mL) pure vanilla extract (optional)

1 tbsp (15 mL) coconut oil

¼ cup (60 mL) coconut butter

3 tbsp (45 mL) real maple syrup or liquid honey

Place oats in a food processor or blender and blend until a flour consistency. Transfer to a large bowl, then add water, ¾ cup (175 mL) of the strawberries, banana, egg and vanilla, if using. Stir until smooth. The pancake batter will be thick.

Melt coconut oil in a large skillet over medium heat. Pour about ¼ cup (60 mL) batter into the pan for each pancake. Cook for 3 to 4 minutes, until bottom of pancake is golden brown, then flip and cook for another few minutes, until bottom is golden brown.

Serve topped with the remaining strawberries, coconut butter and maple syrup or honey.

*If you want this recipe to be truly gluten-free, be sure to purchase certified gluten-free oats, or substitute with quinoa flakes.

Joyous Tip

• • •

I add the egg for extra protein, B₁₂ and iron, but if you can't eat eggs or choose not to, you could always use an egg substitute such as chia. For a step-by-step video of this recipe, visit joyoushealth.com/minipancakes

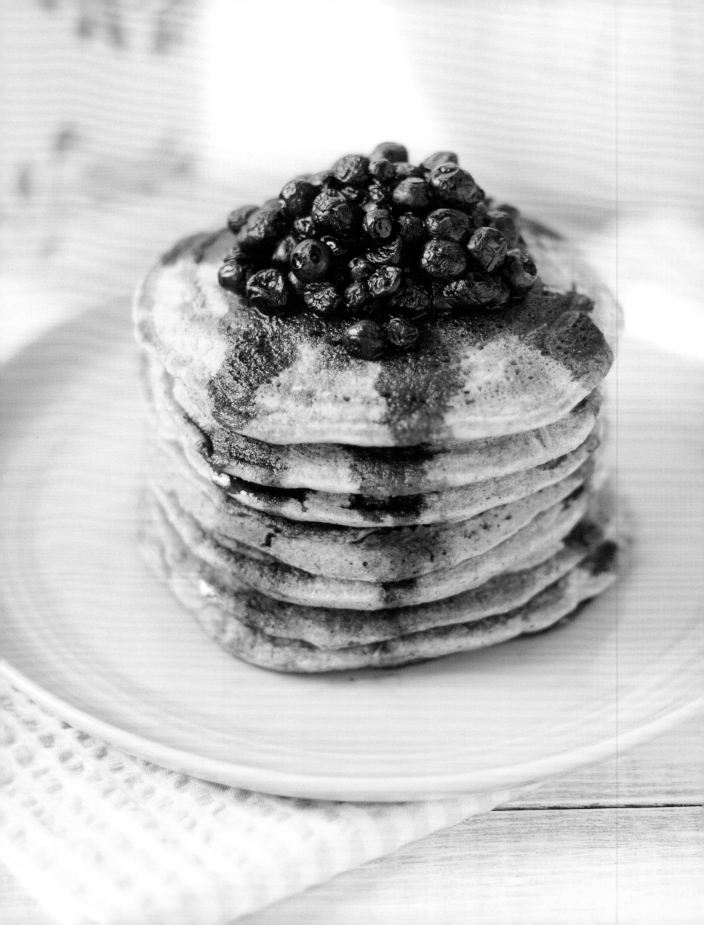

Buckwheat Pancakes with Warmed Blueberries

Buckwheat flour is a gluten-free kitchen essential. I love the fluffiness of these pancakes. If you make extra, you can pop them in the toaster during the week for a quick and healthy gourmet breakfast.

Makes 12 to 14 pancakes

 Vegetarian **Gluten-free** **Dairy-free** **Refined Sugar-free**

1 banana, mashed

2 medium eggs, whisked

1³/₄ cups (425 mL) unsweetened almond milk

1 tsp (5 mL) almond extract

1¹/₂ cups (375 mL) light buckwheat flour

1¹/₂ tsp (7 mL) baking powder

¹/₂ tsp (2 mL) sea salt

1 tbsp (15 mL) coconut oil

Topping

¹/₂ cup (125 mL) fresh or thawed frozen blueberries

1 tbsp (15 mL) filtered water

Real maple syrup (optional)

In a medium bowl, combine banana, eggs, almond milk and almond extract. In a large bowl, whisk together buckwheat flour, baking powder and sea salt. Stir wet ingredients into dry ingredients, then let sit for a few minutes.

Melt coconut oil in a large skillet over medium heat. Pour about ¼ cup (60 mL) batter into the pan for each pancake. Cook for 2 to 3 minutes, until soft bubbles form on top, then flip and cook for another minute or two.

While the pancakes are cooking, combine blueberries and water in a small pot over low heat. Using a fork, press down on the blueberries to break some of them open and release the juices. Heat just until warm.

Spoon blueberries over pancakes and top with maple syrup, if using.

> ## Joyous Tip
> • • •
> If you use thawed frozen berries, be sure to drain them well to remove any excess moisture. You could use dark buckwheat flour, but I recommend light flour. Light is a finer texture compared to dark and it yields a fluffier pancake.

Creamy Comforting Millet Porridge

Millet is a wonderful gluten-free alternative to quinoa and a nice change from oats. You can enjoy it with any fresh fruit you have on hand and top it with your favourite superfoods such as pumpkin seeds or hemp seeds.

Makes 2 servings

 Vegan   Gluten-free   Dairy-free   Refined Sugar-free

½ cup (125 mL) uncooked millet

1 cup (250 mL) filtered water

½ cup (125 mL) unsweetened almond milk

1 tsp (5 mL) ground cinnamon

1 tsp (5 mL) pure vanilla extract

3 tbsp (45 mL) raisins

In a medium pot over high heat, bring millet and water to a boil. Reduce to a simmer for 20 minutes and cover pot with a lid. At 20 minutes add almond milk, cinnamon, vanilla and raisins. Cook for another 5 to 10 minutes until millet is fluffy. If millet seems dry, feel free to add ¼ cup (60 mL) more almond milk.

Top with your choice of any of the following: fresh fruit, nuts and seeds.

Chicken Pesto Frittata

My hubby and I often make this when we're entertaining for brunch because it's always a hit. If I'm lucky enough to have leftovers, I always enjoy it for lunch the next day with a big green salad. This frittata goes well with the Superfood Salad with Creamy Dressing on page 201 or the Purple and Green Cabbage Slaw on page 204.

Makes 4 servings

 Gluten-free   **Dairy-free**   **Sugar-free**

Pesto

2 cups (500 mL) torn kale (centre stems removed)
    or arugula

⅓ cup (75 mL) shelled hemp seeds

½ cup (125 mL) fresh basil (or 2 tsp/10 mL dried)

⅓ cup (75 mL) raw walnuts or almonds

1 to 2 garlic cloves

Juice of ½ lemon

¼ cup (60 mL) extra-virgin olive oil

Frittata

1 tbsp (15 mL) grapeseed oil

1 lb (450 g) boneless, skinless chicken breasts,
    cut into 1-inch (2.5 cm) pieces

½ white onion, thinly sliced

8 to 10 large eggs

⅓ cup (75 mL) unsweetened rice milk or almond milk

1 cup (250 mL) shredded dairy-free cheese

½ cup (125 mL) drained oil-packed sun-dried
    tomatoes, finely chopped

Preheat oven to 400°F (200°C).

To make the pesto, combine all ingredients in a food processor or blender. Process until smooth. Set aside.

To make the frittata, heat grapeseed oil in 10-inch (25 cm) ovenproof skillet over medium heat. Add chicken and cook, stirring frequently, for 5 minutes. Add onions and cook, stirring frequently, for another 2 minutes.

Meanwhile, in a medium bowl, whisk together eggs, rice milk, half of the cheese, sun-dried tomatoes and ⅓ cup (75 mL) of the pesto. Pour egg mixture into skillet and sprinkle remaining cheese on top. Cook, without stirring, for 3 minutes. Transfer skillet to oven and bake for 10 to 12 minutes or until golden brown and a knife inserted in the centre comes out clean. Slice into wedges and top with remaining pesto and your favourite salsa.

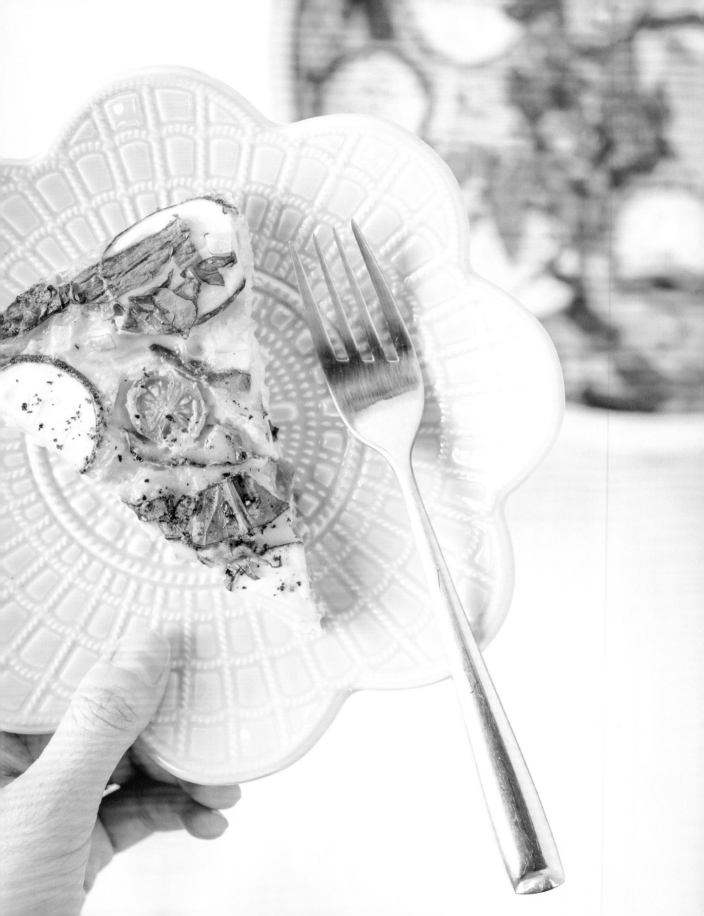

Family Veggie Frittata

This is not your traditional frittata with heavy cream made in a cast-iron skillet. But that's exactly what inspired this recipe! One day while drooling over the photos in one of my favourite food magazines, I decided to whip up this frittata. It was so good I've made it countless times since.

Makes 4 servings

 Vegetarian   Gluten-free   Dairy-free   Sugar-free

8 large eggs

½ cup (125 mL) unsweetened almond milk
    or filtered water

1 tbsp (15 mL) grapeseed oil

2 to 3 garlic cloves, minced

½ red onion, finely chopped

½ cup (125 mL) grape or cherry tomatoes, halved

½ zucchini, thinly sliced

⅓ cup (75 mL) loosely packed chopped fresh basil

½ cup (125 mL) chopped fresh spinach

Sea salt and freshly ground pepper

½ cup (125 mL) shredded dairy-free cheese
    (optional)

Preheat oven to 350°F (180°C). Grease a 10-inch (3 L) round baking dish.

In a large bowl, whisk together eggs and almond milk. Pour into baking dish.

Heat grapeseed oil in a large skillet over medium heat. Add garlic and onions; sauté for a few minutes, until softened. Scrape onion mixture into baking dish and use a spatula to spread it out and mix it in with the egg mixture. Top with tomatoes, zucchini, basil and spinach. Season with sea salt and pepper. If using cheese, sprinkle on top.

Bake for 28 to 30 minutes or until golden brown and a knife inserted in the centre comes out clean. Enjoy with a large green salad.

> ## *Joyous Tip*
> • • •
> When using fresh garlic, be sure to let it sit for 10 minutes after you chop it.
> This allows the health-promoting allicin to form. When garlic is in its whole form,
> a sulphur-based compound called alliin and an enzyme called alliinase are separate.
> Cutting, mincing, chopping or crushing garlic ruptures the cells and allows the enzyme
> to come into contact with the alliin to form a new compound called allicin. It's this
> compound that is responsible for many of the health benefits of garlic.

Coconut Yogurt Parfait with Chia Jam

I consider this my "breakfast of champions" meal! The chia jam and grain-free granola make this parfait fantastic for digestion and will give you a boost of energy for the day. It's also a really nice recipe to make if you are having guests over for brunch because it looks so pretty layered in glasses.

Makes 4 parfaits

 Vegetarian   Gluten-free   Dairy-free   Refined Sugar-free

2 cups (500 mL) plain coconut milk yogurt

1 cup (250 mL) any chia jam (pages 178–179)

2 cups (500 mL) Grain-Free Nutty Granola (page 114)

½ pint (250 mL) fresh blueberries, strawberries or blackberries

2 bananas, sliced

1 to 2 tbsp (15 to 30 mL) liquid honey

Into 4 tall glasses or glass dessert bowls, spoon a large dollop of yogurt, followed by a dollop of chia jam, a spoonful of granola, then some of the fresh berries and banana slices. Drizzle with honey if desired. Repeat the layers in each glass until full.

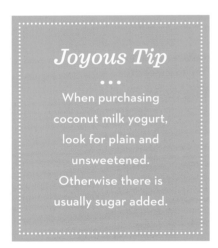

Joyous Tip

• • •

When purchasing coconut milk yogurt, look for plain and unsweetened. Otherwise there is usually sugar added.

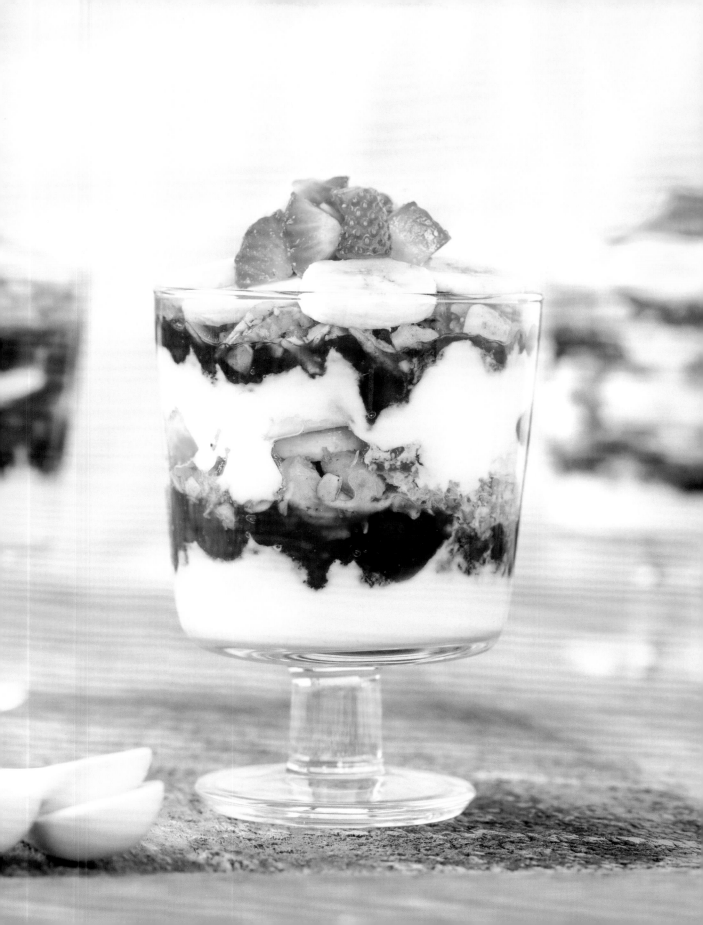

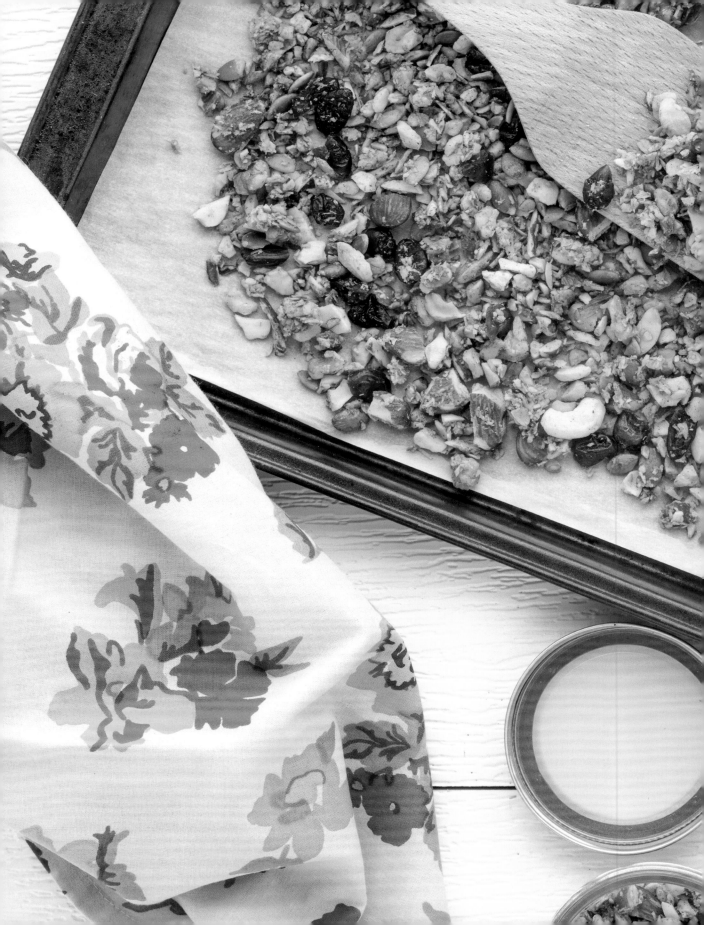

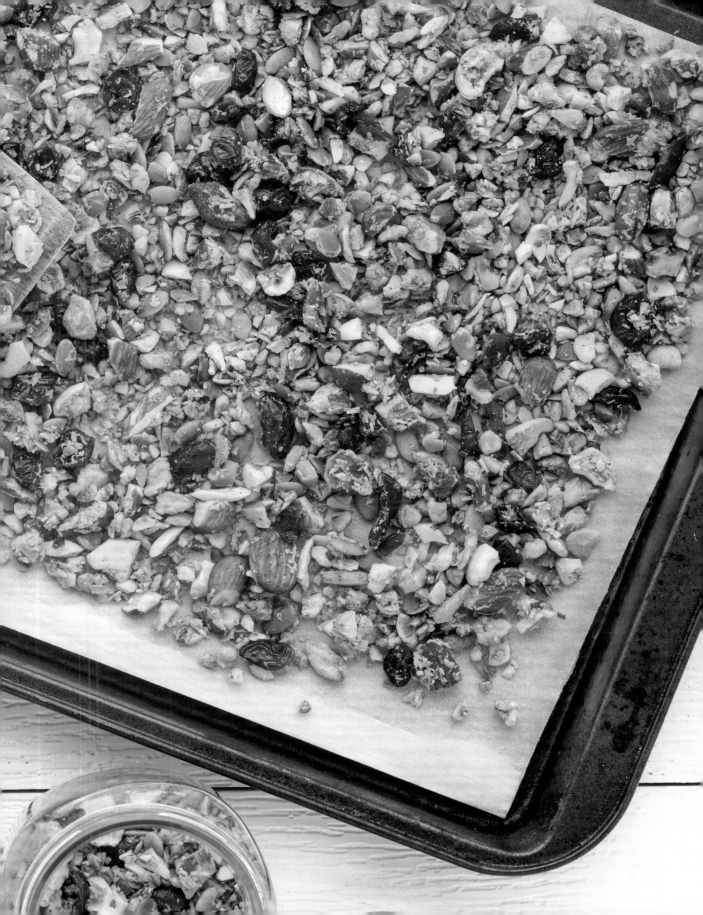

Grain-Free Nutty Granola

I love this granola because the easily digested plant-based protein and good fats in the nuts and seeds make it filling. A little goes a long way—you'll see! Plus, it's completely grain-free, which is wonderful if you have trouble digesting the standard granola grains like oats.

Makes about 8 cups (2 L)

 V Vegan   **GF** Gluten-free   **DF** Dairy-free   **RSF** Refined Sugar-free

4 cups (1 L) mixed raw pecans, cashews and walnuts

1 cup (250 mL) raw pumpkin seeds

1 cup (250 mL) unsweetened, unsulphured shredded coconut

1 cup (250 mL) dried cranberries or dried cherries

1 egg white (optional)

2 tbsp (30 mL) filtered water (optional)

3 tbsp (45 mL) coconut oil, melted

1/3 cup (75 mL) real maple syrup

1 tsp (5 mL) pure vanilla extract or vanilla powder

2 tsp (10 mL) cinnamon

1/2 tsp (2 mL) nutmeg

1/2 tsp (2 mL) sea salt

Preheat oven to 300°F (150°C). Line a baking sheet with parchment paper.

Place nuts and pumpkin seeds in a blender or food processor. Pulse a few times to chop the nuts, but don't grind them into a fine meal. Transfer to a large bowl and stir in coconut and dried cranberries.

In a medium bowl, whisk together egg white with the water, if using, until bubbly and slightly foamy. (You can skip this step if you prefer an egg-free granola. The egg white helps the granola to clump together, but it's not crucial.) Add melted coconut oil, maple syrup, vanilla, cinnamon, nutmeg and sea salt; whisk together well. Pour liquid mixture into nut mixture. Stir everything well to make sure it is all coated.

Spread granola evenly on the baking sheet and bake for 40 minutes, stirring once after 20 minutes, and again at the end. Be careful not to let it burn; it should be golden brown. Let granola cool completely. Transfer to an airtight container, preferably a mason jar.

Joyous Tip

• • •

Many people are sensitive to grains such as oats (even if they are certified gluten-free), and it's very difficult to find a commercial grain-free granola, which is why I created this totally grain-free recipe. This granola can also be beneficial for those with any inflammatory issues such as IBS, who may need to take a break from grains.

Joy's Favourite Breakfast Cookies

I love these cookies! They are packed with fibre, flavour and nutrition. I make batches of them to freeze when I know I'm going to have a super-busy week. I enjoy them straight out of the freezer too. These are the perfect grab-and-go breakfast food or snack. Enjoy with a Refreshing Green Juice on page 149.

Makes 12 to 14 cookies

 Vegetarian   **Gluten-free**   **Dairy-free**   **Refined Sugar-free**

1 cup (250 mL) brown rice flour

³/₄ cup (175 mL) almond meal/flour (ground almonds)

2 tbsp (30 mL) cinnamon

¹/₂ tsp (2 mL) baking soda

1 cup (250 mL) old-fashioned rolled oats

¹/₂ cup (125 mL) raisins

¹/₄ cup (60 mL) ground flaxseeds

¹/₄ cup (60 mL) unsweetened, unsulphured coconut flakes

¹/₄ cup (60 mL) chopped walnuts (optional)

2 large eggs

³/₄ cup (175 mL) coconut oil, melted

¹/₄ cup (60 mL) real maple syrup

2 tbsp (30 mL) blackstrap molasses

1 banana, mashed

1 tsp (5 mL) pure vanilla extract

Preheat oven to 350°F (180°C). Grease a baking sheet with coconut oil or line with parchment paper.

In a large bowl, whisk together brown rice flour, almond flour, cinnamon and baking soda. Stir in oats, raisins, flaxseeds, coconut flakes and walnuts, if using.

In a small bowl, whisk eggs. Whisk in melted coconut oil, maple syrup, molasses, mashed banana and vanilla. Pour into dry mixture and stir just until well combined, but do not overmix.

Drop by large spoonfuls onto the baking sheet and press down lightly with the back of a spoon or with your hand. Bake for 12 to 14 minutes; the edges will be a little browner.

Store in the fridge for up to 10 days. These cookies also freeze well for months.

Joyous Tip

• • •

If you have trouble digesting oats or you are looking for a change, you can make these cookies with 1 cup (250 mL) of quinoa flakes instead of oats. Keep in mind that oats are only truly gluten-free if they are labelled "gluten-free."

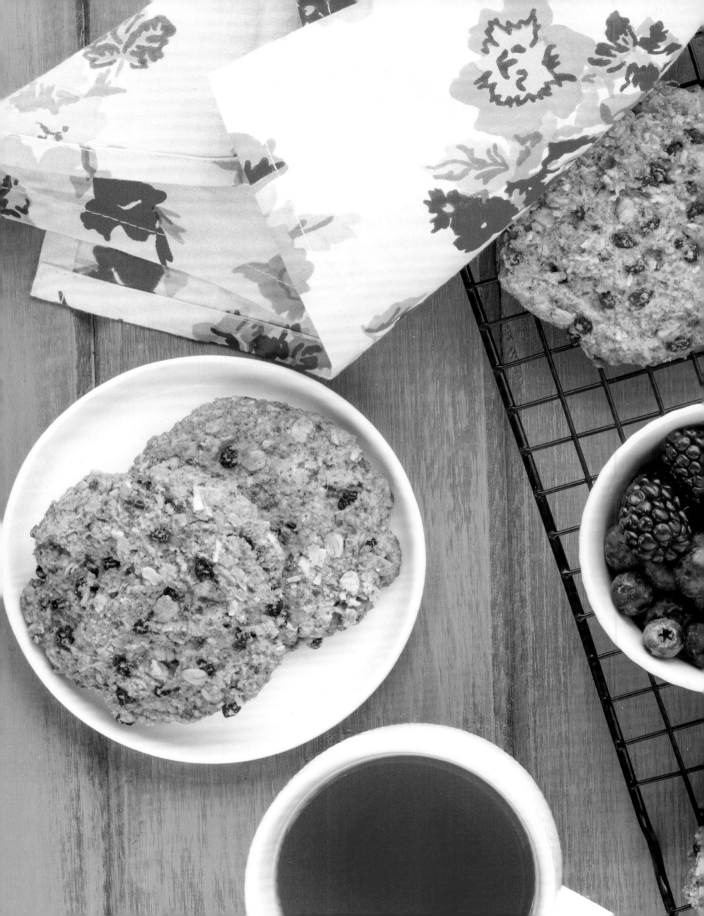

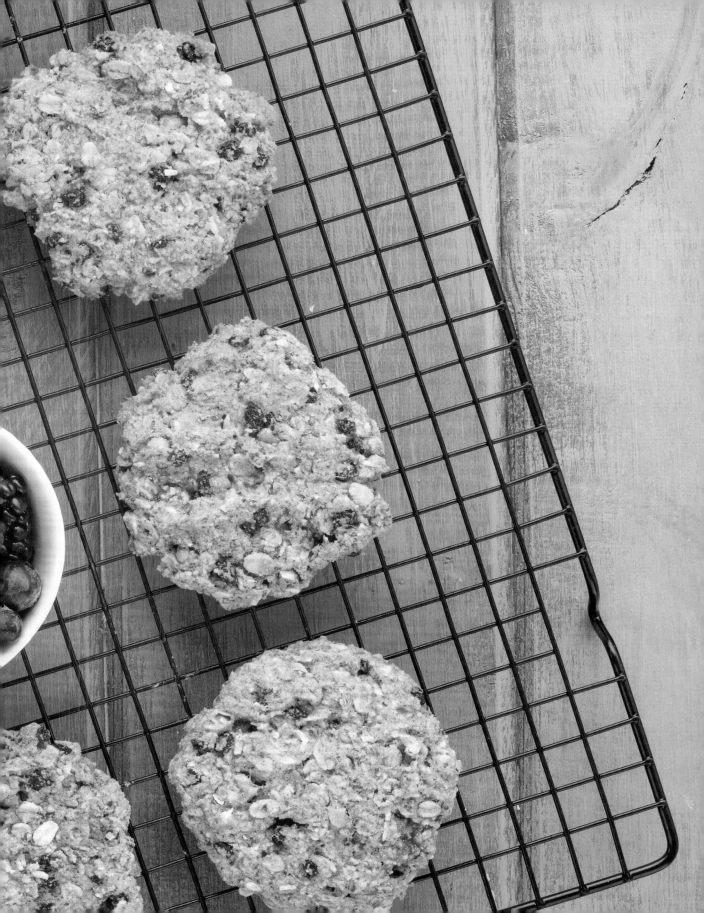

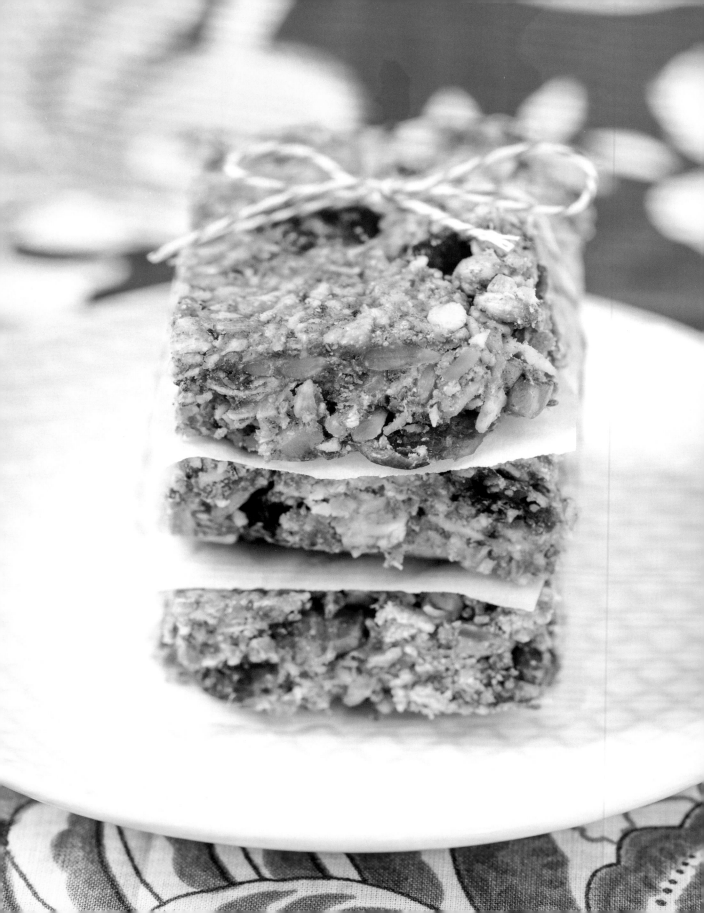

No-Bake Superfood Breakfast Bars

When you don't want to turn on your oven but you want a breakfast bar that is packed with nutrition and super satisfying, these bars are perfect. I also love eating them post-exercise or when I'm on the go. Enjoy with a cup of Detox Ginger Tea on page 131.

Makes 12 bars

 Vegan Gluten-free Dairy-free Sugar-free

1 cup (250 mL) old-fashioned rolled oats

³/₄ cup (175 mL) dried cranberries

³/₄ cup (175 mL) unsweetened, unsulphured shredded coconut

¹/₂ cup (125 mL) raw sunflower seeds

¹/₄ cup (60 mL) chia seeds

1 tbsp (15 mL) cinnamon

1 tsp (5 mL) pure vanilla extract

¹/₂ cup (125 mL) almond butter (or sunflower seed butter for a nut-free option)

2 bananas, mashed

Zest of 1 organic orange

¹/₂ cup (125 mL) vanilla, chocolate or natural-flavour protein powder

¹/₄ cup (60 mL) coconut oil, melted

Combine all ingredients in a large bowl and mix well. Press into a 9-inch (2.5 L) square pan and refrigerate for 4 hours. Cut into squares and enjoy. Store in the fridge or freezer.

Joyous Tip

• • •

Since these bars aren't baked, you don't need to worry about the size of pan. The smaller the pan, the thicker the bar, and the larger the pan, the thinner the bar. It's up to you!

Guacamole Devilled Eggs

I have such fond memories of my grandma's devilled eggs. Every special family gathering like Easter, she would make them for us. I've combined two of my favourite recipes—guacamole and devilled eggs—into one devilishly good breakfast, appetizer or side dish. If you have some leftover guac-devilled egg paste, enjoy it with crackers, on toast or as a dip for veggies.

Makes 8 devilled eggs

 Vegetarian   Gluten-free   Dairy-free **SF** Sugar-free

4 medium or large organic eggs, hard-boiled for 8 minutes and cooled

1 ripe avocado, peeled and pitted

1/2 small tomato, finely chopped

1 garlic clove, finely chopped

2 tbsp (30 mL) finely chopped red onion

2 tbsp (30 mL) finely chopped fresh cilantro

2 tbsp (30 mL) shelled hemp seeds

Juice of 1 lime

Pinch of cayenne pepper

Dash of sea salt

Peel the eggs, cut them in half lengthwise and scoop yolks into a medium bowl.

Add avocado to the egg yolks and mash together with a fork. Then stir in tomato, garlic, red onion, cilantro, hemp seeds, lime juice, cayenne and sea salt. Carefully spoon the mixture into each egg white half. Sprinkle with additional cayenne or paprika.

> *Joyous Tip*
>
> • • •
>
> For a step-by-step video of this recipe to follow along with, visit joyoushealth.com/gauceggs.

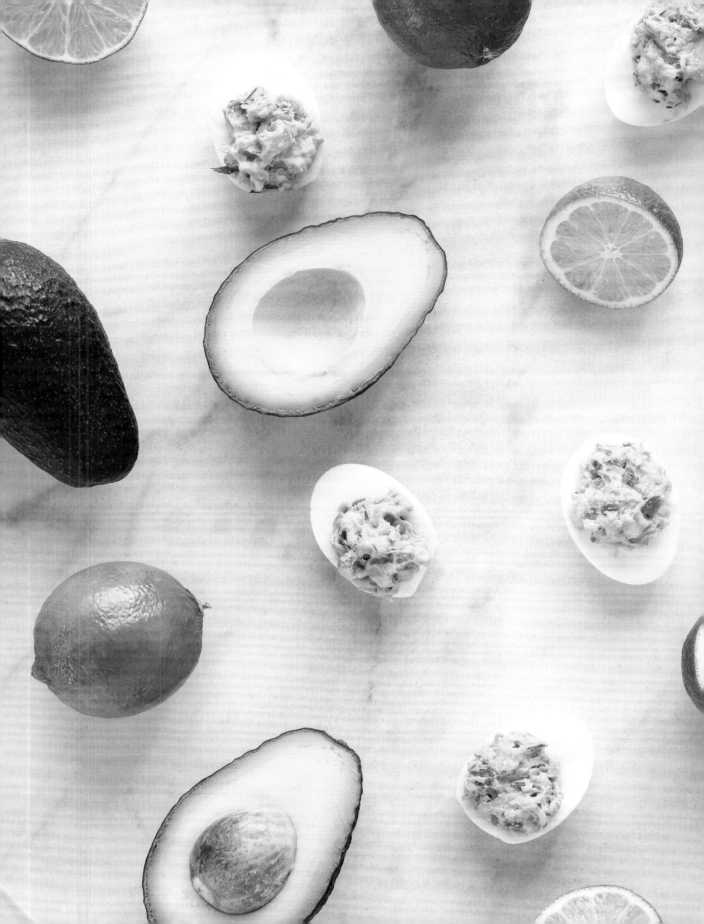

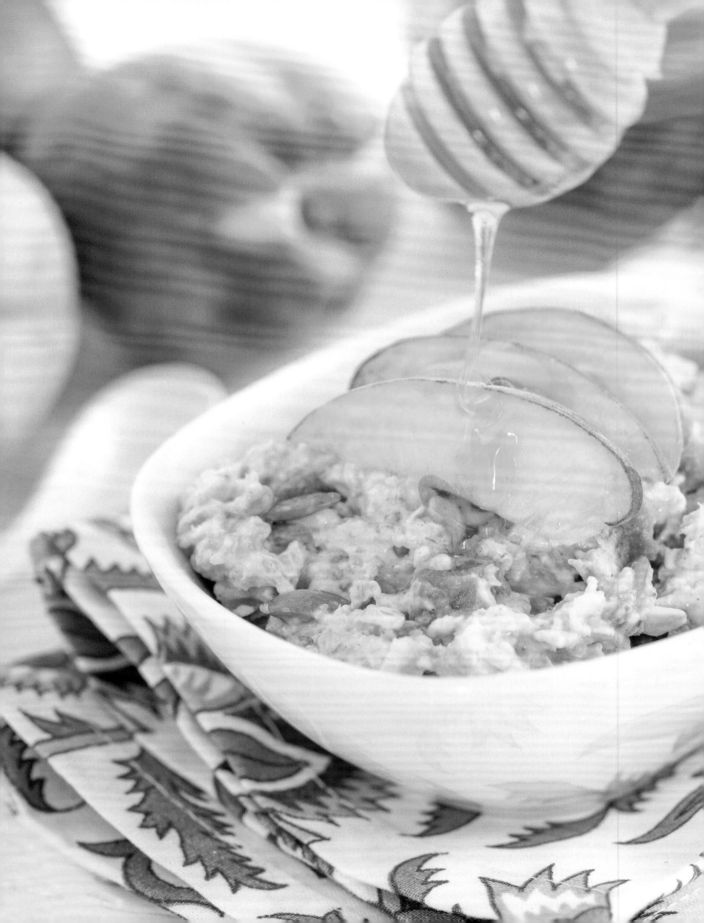

Overnight Oatmeal with Peaches and Apricots

You'll love waking up to this oatmeal because it is the quintessential breakfast comfort food. It is filling because it is full of fibre, plant-based protein and good fat. You'll be able to power through the morning with ease!

Makes 2 to 3 servings

 Vegan   Gluten-free   Dairy-free   Refined Sugar-free

2 cups (500 mL) old-fashioned rolled oats

2 cups (500 mL) unsweetened almond milk

¼ cup (60 mL) chopped dried apricots

3 tbsp (45 mL) chia seeds

2 tbsp (30 mL) raw pumpkin seeds

2 tbsp (30 mL) raw sunflower seeds

1 tsp (5 mL) cinnamon

½ tsp (2 mL) nutmeg

1 peach, pitted and sliced

1 tsp (5 mL) liquid honey (optional)

In a large bowl, combine all ingredients except the peach. Stir well, cover and let sit overnight in fridge.

The next day, spoon desired amount into bowls, add more almond milk if you wish and top with fresh peach slices. Drizzle with honey, if desired.

Cinnamon Toast with Pecan Butter and Chia Jam

My favourite way to enjoy my Best Ever Cinnamon Flaxseed Bread on page 127 is to toast it and spread it with pecan butter and chia jam. This toast is delightful with the Matcha Coconut Milk Latte on page 158.

Makes 1 serving

 Vegetarian   Gluten-free   Dairy-free   Refined Sugar-free

2 slices Best Ever Cinnamon Flaxseed Bread (page 127)

2 tbsp (30 mL) Cinnamon Pecan Butter (page 174)

2 tbsp (30 mL) Blueberry Chia Jam (page 178)

Toast cinnamon bread and top with Cinnamon Pecan Butter followed by Blueberry Chia Jam.

Superfood Quinoa Bowl

This bowl is full of an incredible number of superfoods. It is rich in fibre, vitamins C and B-complex, omega-3s and amino acids and is bursting with antioxidants from all those gorgeous coloured plant pigments. If you have leftover quinoa on hand, this comes together in a snap.

Makes 2 servings

 Vegan   Gluten-free   Dairy-free   Refined Sugar-free

1 cup (250 mL) cooked white quinoa

2 bananas, sliced

1/2 cup (125 mL) strawberries, chopped

1/4 cup (60 mL) pecan halves

1/2 cup (125 mL) blackberries

1/4 cup (60 mL) blueberries

2 tsp (10 mL) chia seeds

1/2 tsp (2 mL) cinnamon

2 tbsp (30 mL) raw pumpkin seeds

Drizzle of liquid honey (optional)

You have two options for putting this together. The simplest way is to combine all the ingredients in a large bowl, then divide between 2 cereal bowls.

For a layered look, divide the ingredients in half and assemble as follows in 2 cereal bowls: Place quinoa in bowls, then layer from the outside to the inside with banana, strawberries, pecans, blackberries and blueberries. Sprinkle with chia seeds, cinnamon and pumpkin seeds, then drizzle with honey. Enjoy with 1/2 to 1 cup (125 to 250 mL) almond milk or a few dollops of coconut yogurt if you like.

> ## *Joyous Tip*
> • • •
> If you've ever had trouble making the perfect quinoa, you're not alone. The trick to quinoa is to make sure you cook it long enough for it to get fluffy. This means cook it until the outside ring separates from the grain of the quinoa. Check out my video on how to make the fluffiest quinoa ever on my Joyous Health YouTube channel, joyoushealth1.
> Quinoa is an excellent source of easily digested plant-based protein. Protein fuels your metabolic rate and keeps you satisfied.

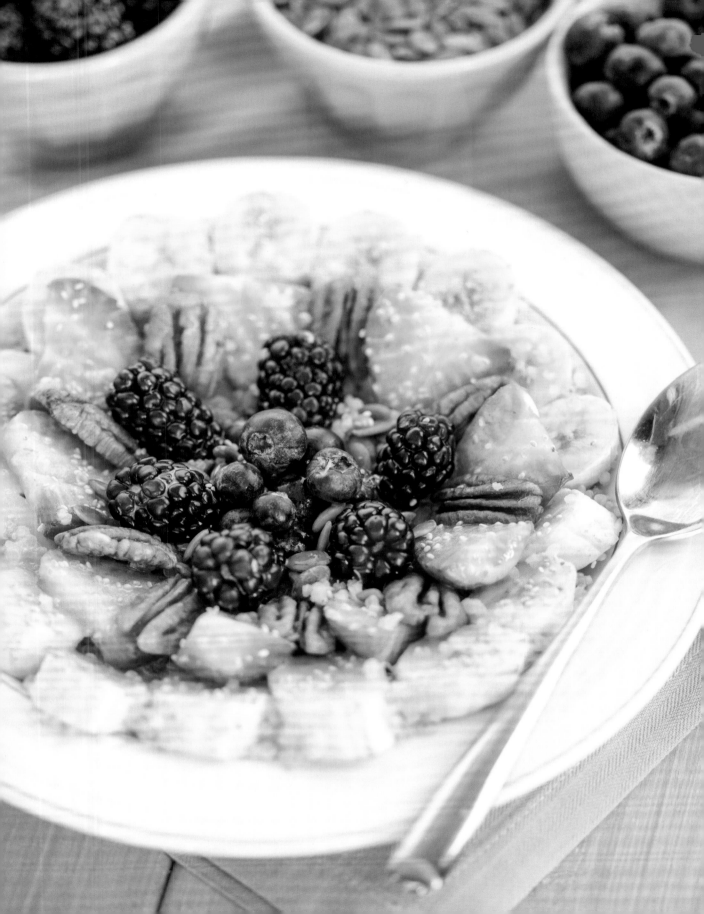

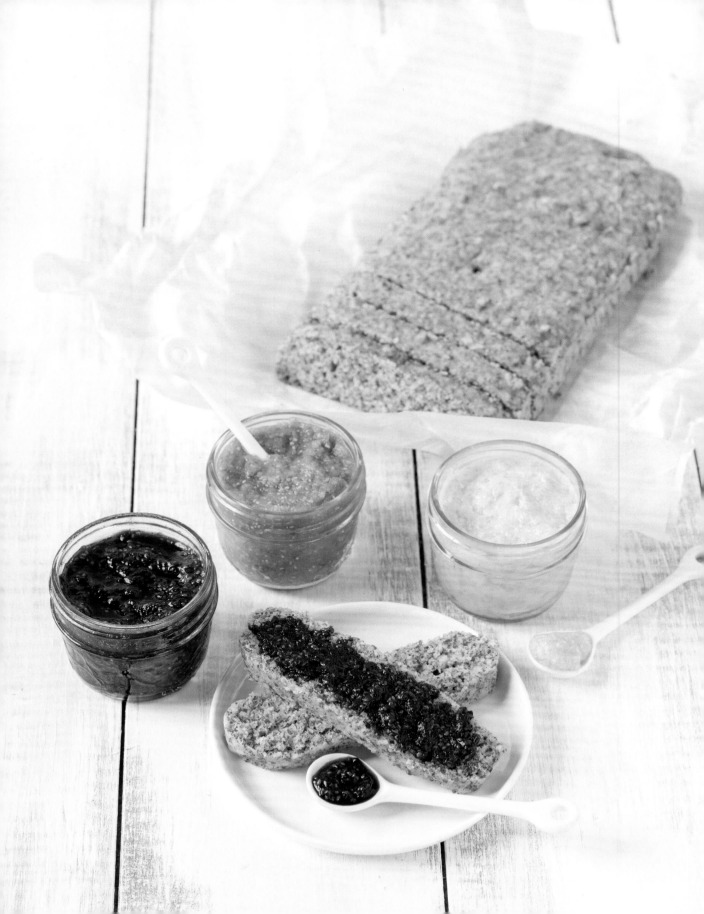

Best Ever Cinnamon Flaxseed Bread

There are many delicious gluten-free breads on the market now, but the problem with many of them is the large number of ingredients. This bread is made of simple whole-food ingredients you can easily find. I enjoy it with Cinnamon Pecan Butter on page 174 and chia jam on pages 178–179.

Makes 1 loaf

 Vegetarian   Gluten-free   Dairy-free   Sugar-free

1 cup (250 mL) almond meal/flour (ground almonds)

⅓ cup (75 mL) chickpea flour

⅔ cup (150 mL) ground flaxseeds

1½ tsp (7 mL) baking powder

1 tsp (5 mL) cinnamon

½ tsp (2 mL) sea salt

4 medium eggs

¼ cup (60 mL) unsweetened almond milk

3 tbsp (45 mL) coconut oil, melted

Preheat oven to 350°F (180°C). Line a loaf pan with parchment paper or grease with coconut oil. (You can use whatever size pan you have handy. A standard 9- by 5-inch/2 L pan will yield a taller loaf than the one in the photo.) If using parchment paper, leave some overhang on the sides to easily lift out the baked bread.

In a large bowl, combine almond flour, chickpea flour, ground flaxseeds, baking powder, cinnamon and sea salt. In a separate bowl, whisk together eggs, almond milk and coconut oil. Stir wet ingredients into dry just until mixed. Do not overmix. The batter will be thick.

Turn batter into the loaf pan. Using a spatula, even out the batter in the pan. Bake for 20 to 22 minutes or until a toothpick inserted in the centre comes out clean. Cool for 10 minutes before removing from the pan and cooling completely on a wire rack. Bread keeps in the fridge for up to a week.

Joyous Tip

• • •

You can freeze this loaf and it will keep for months. Slice it before freezing, so you can pull out a slice or two whenever you wish. Pop a frozen slice directly into the toaster.

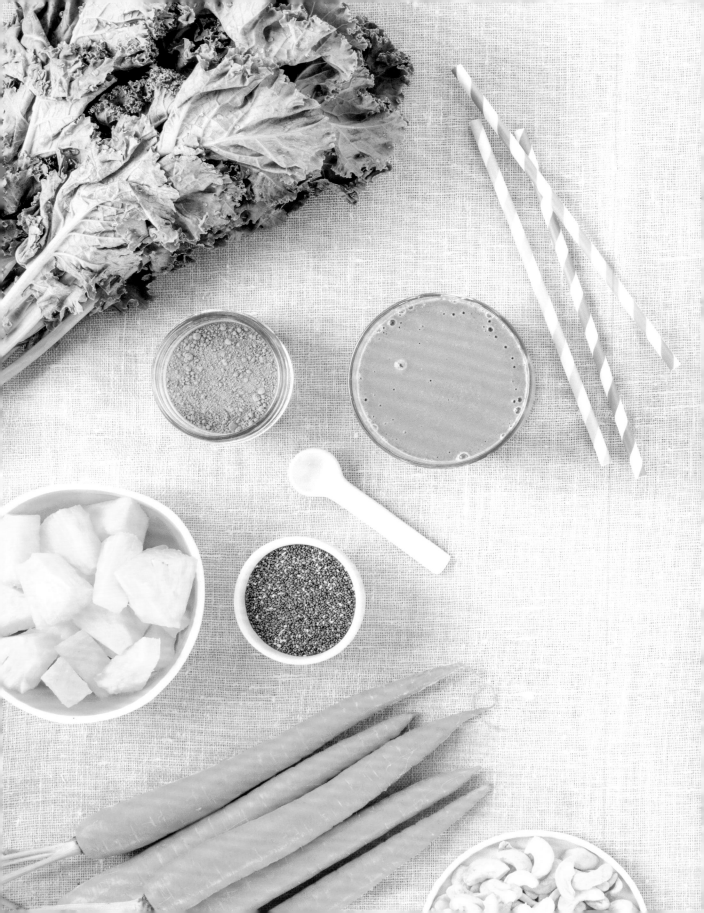

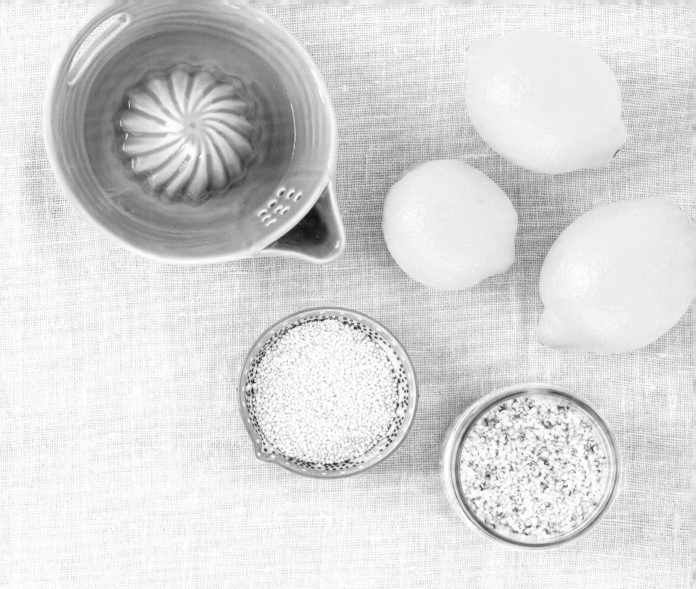

STRAWS and SPOONS

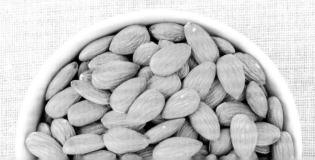

Detox Ginger Tea

Aside from the obvious detox benefits of this tea, it is perfect for many different reasons. These include supporting your immune system if you're coming down with a cold, warming you up on a chilly day or giving your digestive system a little love.

Makes 1 serving

 Vegan   Gluten-free   Dairy-free   Sugar-free

1½ cups (375 mL) filtered water

1 large chunk of ginger root (or 2 tbsp/30 mL grated fresh ginger)

Juice of ½ lemon

Pinch of cayenne pepper (optional)

Boil the water. Pour boiling water into a large mug. Add ginger and lemon, and let steep for 5 minutes. Add a pinch of cayenne if you like.

Drink on an empty stomach at the start of the day or any time you feel like it.

> ## *Joyous Tip*
> • • •
> You might be wondering, why cayenne? Capsaicin is the active ingredient in cayenne and it is a stimulant for both the circulatory and digestive systems. Increased circulation aids lymphatic drainage, meaning more efficient detox, and also gets the gastric juices flowing. Capsaicin is also an anti-inflammatory, and it helps to suppress your appetite, which can be beneficial if you are prone to overeating.

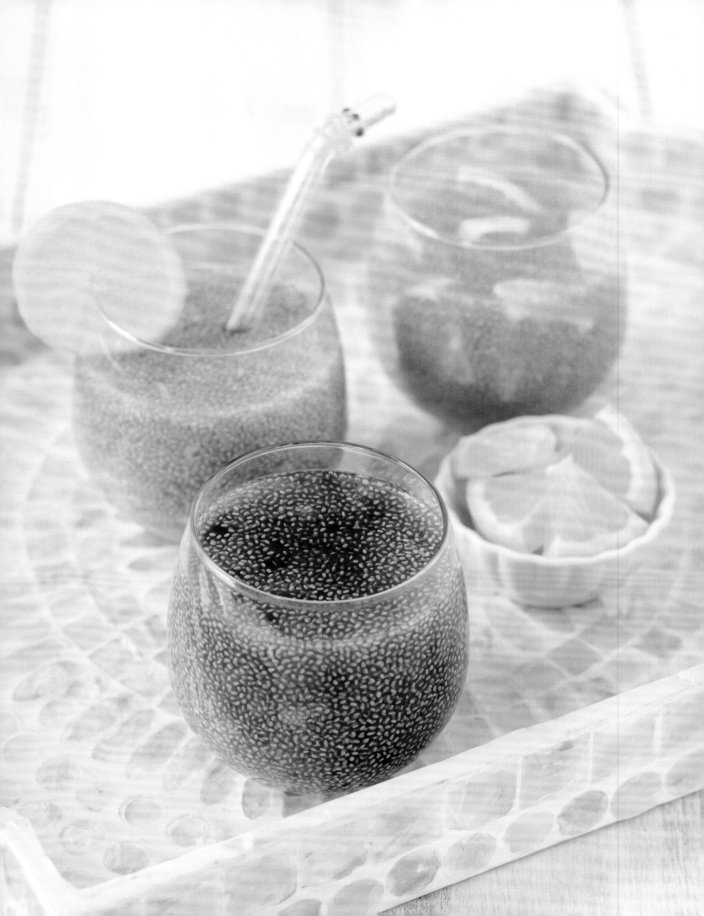

Chia Seed Blueberry Drink

Mainly because of its high fibre content, chia is a detox superfood. All that fibre not only will get things going, so to speak, but will expand in your belly, keeping you fuller longer. This drink makes a great snack between meals.

Makes 2 servings

 V Vegan   **GF** Gluten-free   **DF** Dairy-free   **SF** Sugar-free

2 tbsp (30 mL) chia seeds
1 cup (250 mL) filtered water
1 cup (250 mL) coconut water
1/4 cup (60 mL) fresh or thawed frozen blueberries

Stir chia into 1/2 cup (125 mL) of the water. Let sit in the fridge overnight. In the morning, combine with remaining water, coconut water and blueberries.

Chia Seed Orange Kombucha

This drink is incredible for digestion, combining the high fibre content of chia seeds with kombucha, a fermented tea beverage rich in good bacteria. You can find kombucha at your local health food store.

Makes 2 servings

 V Vegan   **GF** Gluten-free   **DF** Dairy-free   **SF** Sugar-free

2 tbsp (30 mL) chia seeds
1 cup (250 mL) filtered water
1/2 orange, sliced
1 cup (250 mL) kombucha

Stir chia into 1/2 cup (125 mL) of the water, then add orange slices. Let sit in the fridge overnight. In the morning, combine with remaining water and kombucha.

Chia Seed Ginger Lemon Drink

Ginger is a wonderful anti-inflammatory food, and lemon is a fantastic natural detoxifier. These two ingredients combined with the fibre in chia seeds make this the ultimate detox drink.

Makes 2 servings

V Vegan **GF** Gluten-free **DF** Dairy-free **SF** Sugar-free

2 tbsp (30 mL) chia seeds

2 cups (500 mL) filtered water

½ tsp (2 mL) grated fresh ginger

Juice of 1 lemon

Stir chia into ½ cup (125 mL) of the water. Let sit in the fridge overnight. In the morning, combine with remaining water, ginger and lemon juice.

Daily Detox Zinger Elixir

An elixir is a magical or medicinal potion. I had my first one years ago, at a beautiful yoga studio in Florida. Before every yoga class, I would dig into their fridge for an elixir shot prior to my practice, and then enjoy a fresh raw juice afterward, like the Green Sparkle Juice on page 152.

Makes 6 to 7 servings

 Vegan Gluten-free Dairy-free Sugar-free

2 lemons, rind and seeds removed

2 thumb-size chunks peeled fresh ginger

1/2 cup (125 mL) fresh pineapple chunks

1/4 tsp (1 mL) cayenne pepper

1/4 tsp (1 mL) turmeric

Filtered water, just enough for desired consistency

Place all ingredients except water in a blender and pulse until smooth, adding water as needed. Drink a 2-oz (60 mL) shot at a time. Refrigerate up to 2 days or freeze for a week.

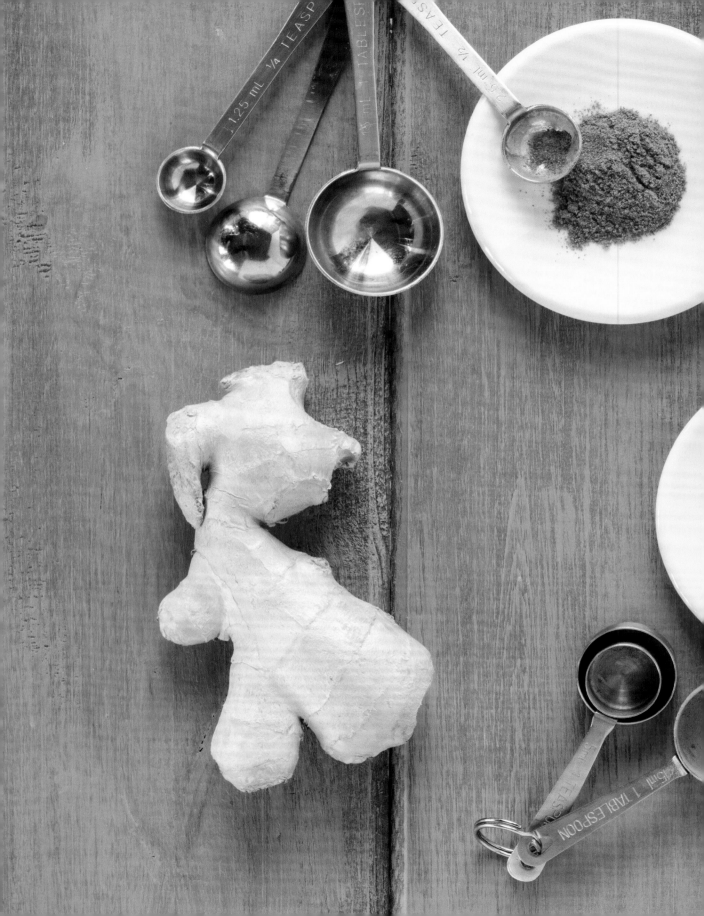

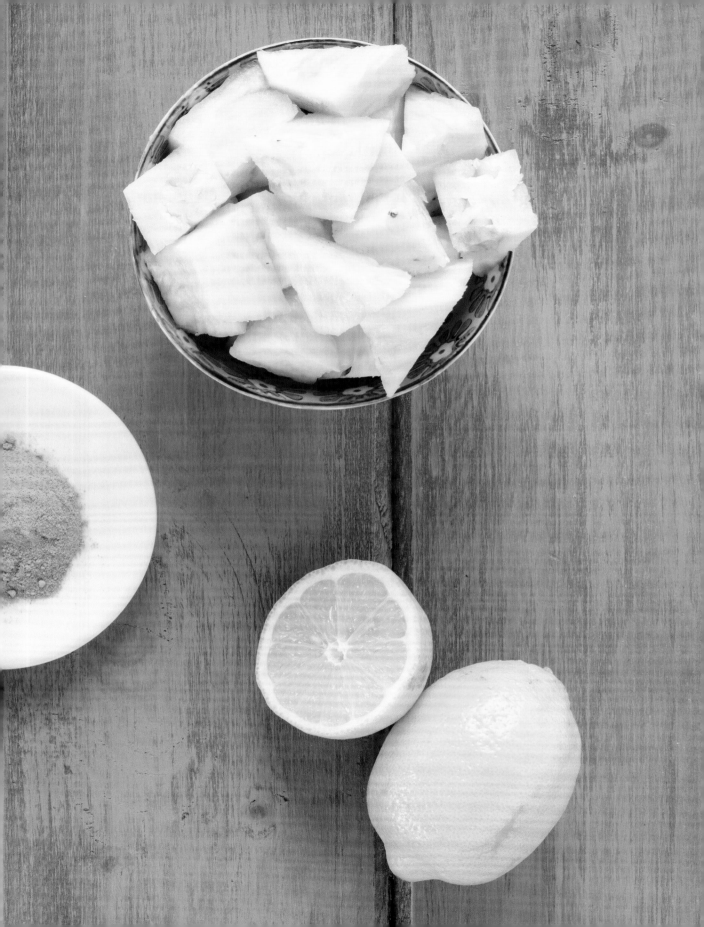

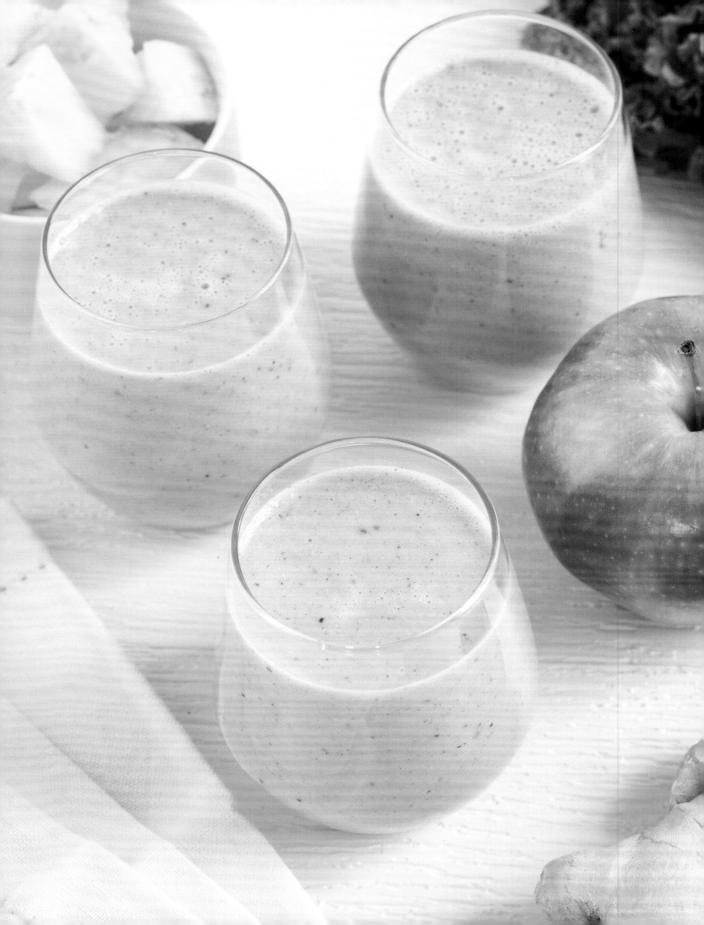

Green Sparkle Smoothie

Once of the best ways to get glowing and sparkling is to eat foods that are detoxifying and thereby beautifying. This smoothie will definitely help you glow from the inside out!

Makes 1 or 2 smoothies

 Vegan **GF** **Gluten-free** **DF** **Dairy-free** **SF** **Sugar-free**

½ banana

1 apple, cut in half and cored

1 cup (250 mL) loosely packed torn fresh kale

¾ cup (175 mL) fresh or frozen pineapple chunks

¼ cup (60 mL) shelled hemp seeds

1 tbsp (15 mL) grated fresh ginger

1½ cups (375 mL) coconut water

Filtered water, just enough for desired consistency

Place all ingredients except water in a blender. Blend for 30 to 60 seconds, until smooth, adding water as needed.

Joyous Tip

• • •

It is best to enjoy smoothies immediately to get the most out of their nutritional value. This is especially true for the enzymes, as they die quickly. You may want to consider purchasing organic for foods that have the highest pesticide residues, like apples.

Apple Spice Smoothie

With the natural sweetness of its ingredients, this smoothie could easily be a dessert. Every time I drink it, these spices remind me of apple pie.

Makes 1 smoothie

 Vegan　 Gluten-free　 Dairy-free　 Sugar-free

1 banana

1 Medjool date, pitted

2 dried or fresh figs

3 to 4 tbsp (45 to 60 mL) vanilla plant-based protein powder

2 tbsp (30 mL) shelled hemp seeds

½ tsp (2 mL) cinnamon

¼ tsp (1 mL) nutmeg

1 cup (250 mL) nut milk of your choice

Filtered water, just enough for desired consistency

Place all ingredients except water in a blender. Blend for 30 to 60 seconds, until smooth, adding water as needed.

> *Joyous Tip*
>
> • • •
>
> I highly recommend you make your own nut milk—see page 148. It is the best way to avoid unnecessary additives, and it tastes far better too.
> If you only have a plain protein powder, add ½ tsp (2 mL) pure vanilla extract.
> Be sure to use a protein powder that contains at least 15 to 20 g of protein, to help balance your blood sugar. If you are new to protein powder, start out with half the amount the first time until you get used to the flavour.
> Be sure to buy a high-quality protein powder, as unfortunately there are a lot of junk protein products on the market.

Joyous Energy Smoothie

When I was pregnant I would totally crave this creamy smoothie. I called it my "bean machine" smoothie! It is incredibly nourishing and energizing with all its vitamins, minerals and antioxidants, and it's super tasty too.

Makes 1 smoothie

 Vegan   **Gluten-free**   **Dairy-free**   **Sugar-free**

¾ cup (175 mL) frozen raspberries

¼ cup (60 mL) raw cashews

¼ to ½ ripe avocado, peeled and pitted

Approximately 1 tbsp (15 mL) superfood mixed berry and green powder

3 to 4 tbsp (45 to 60 mL) plant-based protein powder (any flavour)

1 tbsp (15 mL) chia seeds

1 cup (250 mL) unsweetened almond or coconut milk

Filtered water, just enough for desired consistency

Place all ingredients except water in a blender. Blend for 30 to 60 seconds, until smooth, adding water as needed.

Joyous Tip

• • •

You can find a variety of superfood vegetable and fruit powders at health food stores and online. Choose one that is well researched and does not contain unnecessary ingredients. Every ingredient should have a purpose. I used a superfood mixed berry and green powder that was safe for pregnancy. Many of these powders contain herbs that are not safe if you are pregnant, so be sure to read the labels carefully. If you're still not sure, ask your natural healthcare practitioner.

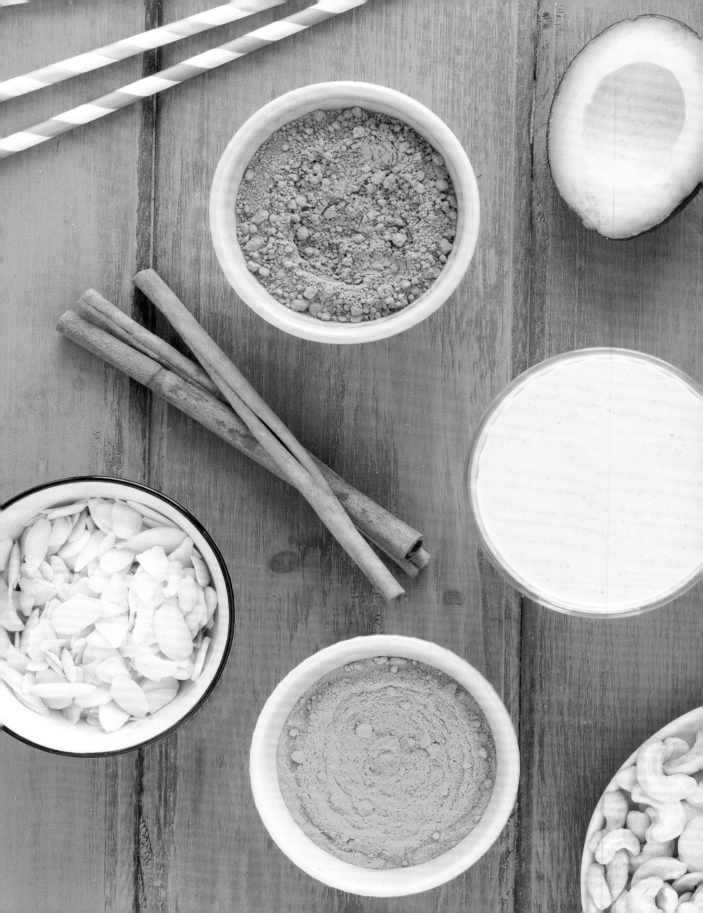

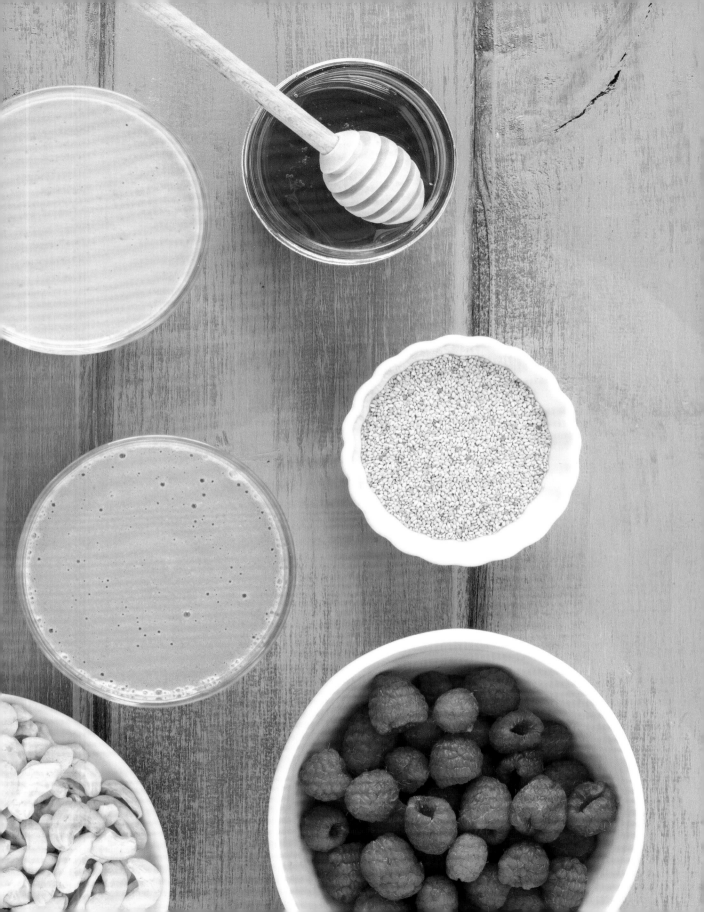

Soothing Golden Smoothie

This smoothie is super packed with anti-inflammatory and detoxifying superfood ingredients such as turmeric and ginger. The cinnamon balances blood sugar and is delicious too. This is the perfect dessert smoothie, but I won't tell if you enjoy it for breakfast.

Makes 1 smoothie

 Vegan Gluten-free Dairy-free Sugar-free

⅓ cup (75 mL) unsweetened, unsulphured coconut flakes

3 tbsp (45 mL) shelled hemp seeds

1 tsp (5 mL) cinnamon

½ tsp (2 mL) turmeric

2 tsp (10 mL) grated fresh ginger (or 1 tsp/5 mL ground)

3 large Medjool dates, pitted, or 1 banana

1 tbsp (15 mL) coconut butter

Coconut milk, just enough for desired consistency

Place all ingredients in a blender. Blend for 30 to 60 seconds, until smooth, adding more coconut milk as needed.

Matcha Green Tea Smoothie

Matcha is a detox superfood and provides a "clean" energy, unlike coffee. It is extremely high in antioxidants, more so than green tea, blueberries or even red wine. The raw honey does a nice job at softening the distinct flavour of the matcha, especially if you are not used to the taste.

Makes 1 smoothie

 Vegetarian Gluten-free Dairy-free Refined Sugar-free

1 banana

1/2 ripe avocado, peeled and pitted

3 to 4 tbsp (45 to 60 mL) vanilla plant-based protein powder

1 tbsp (15 mL) raw honey

1 tsp (5 mL) matcha green tea powder

1 cup (250 mL) nut milk of your choice

Filtered water, just enough for desired consistency

Place all ingredients except water in a blender. Blend for 30 to 60 seconds, until smooth, adding water as needed.

> *Joyous Tip*
>
> • • •
>
> If you have only a plain protein powder, simply add 1/2 tsp (2 mL) pure vanilla extract. You can find matcha powder at specialty tea shops and health food stores. Be sure to buy "shade-grown" and preferably certified organic matcha powder.

Rejuvenate Me Smoothie

As the name suggests, this smoothie is incredibly rejuvenating. It is packed with protein from the spirulina, hemp and protein powder. It is also full of detoxifying plant compounds, including chlorophyll, fibre and antioxidants.

Makes 1 to 2 smoothies

 Vegan   Gluten-free   Dairy-free   Sugar-free

1 cup (250 mL) firmly packed fresh spinach

$^1/_2$ cup (125 mL) loosely packed fresh mint leaves

1 apple (unpeeled if organic), cored and cut into pieces

$^1/_2$ cup (125 mL) fresh or frozen pineapple chunks

$^1/_2$ lime, peel removed

$^1/_4$ cup (60 mL) shelled hemp seeds

$^1/_2$ tsp (2 mL) spirulina powder

3 to 4 tbsp (45 to 60 mL) plant-based protein powder (optional)

Filtered water or coconut water, just enough for desired consistency

Place all ingredients except water in a blender. Blend for 30 to 60 seconds, until smooth, adding water as needed.

> ### *Joyous Tip*
> • • •
> Spirulina is a blue-green alga that can be purchased in powder form at your local health food store. It is rich in iron, copper and B vitamins and it is a rich source of chlorophyll, making it a wonderfully detoxifying food.

Blueberry Bliss Smoothie Bowl

Have you ever made a smoothie too thick to drink? That's exactly what happened to me once, so I decided to enjoy it with a spoon! Then it morphed into a breakfast bowl because I started adding my grain-free granola for some crunch. Fulfilling, detox friendly and yummy!

Makes 1 to 2 servings

 Vegan   Gluten-free   Dairy-free   Sugar-free

½ ripe avocado, peeled and pitted

1 banana

¾ cup (175 mL) fresh or frozen strawberries, raspberries or blueberries

3 to 4 tbsp (45 to 60 mL) plant-based protein powder

1 cup (250 mL) Nutty Milk (page 148)

Ice, for desired consistency

½ cup (125 mL) Grain-Free Nutty Granola (page 114)

2 tbsp (30 mL) unsweetened, unsulphured coconut flakes, for garnish

Place all ingredients except granola and coconut flakes in a blender. Blend for 30 to 60 seconds, until smooth, adding more ice as needed. Pour into a bowl and top with granola and coconut flakes.

Nutty Milk

This homemade nut milk will take all your smoothies to the next level. Not only does it taste amazing compared to store-bought but you don't have to worry about any added sugar, sodium or unnecessary additives.

Makes about 5 cups (1.25 L)

 Vegan   **GF** **Gluten-free**   **DF** **Dairy-free**   **SF** **Sugar-free**

1 cup (250 mL) raw cashews, brazil nuts, hazelnuts, almonds, pecans or walnuts

4 cups (1 L) filtered water, plus more for soaking nuts

½ tsp (2 mL) vanilla powder

Pinch of sea salt

Soak nuts in water to cover for 4 to 6 hours. Drain and rinse well.

In a blender combine nuts, vanilla powder, sea salt and 4 cups (1 L) water. Blend until you can no longer see any chunks of nuts. Strain through a fine-mesh sieve or nut bag set over a bowl. Nut milk keeps in the fridge for up to 5 days.

> *Joyous Tip*
>
> • • •
>
> You can use the same amount of coconut flakes in place of the nuts. You do not need to soak the coconut flakes ahead of time.

Refreshing Green Juice

Drinking this juice is like hitting the reset button on Monday morning. In the heat of summer it is incredibly hydrating, but any time of year, this juice is refreshing.

Makes 1 to 2 servings

 Vegan Gluten-free Dairy-free **SF** Sugar-free

1 apple

1 pear

¼ cucumber

4 celery stalks

2 kale or romaine lettuce leaves

1 thumb-size piece fresh ginger

Wash all ingredients. Cut fruits and vegetables into small chunks that will fit the mouth of your juice extractor. Remove the seeds from the apple and pear. You may add ¼ cup (60 mL) water to the juice extractor at the end to get every last drop of juice. Enjoy immediately.

> ## *Joyous Tip*
> • • •
> Juicing is a wonderful way to maximize your nutrition, because in one convenient glass you get a concentrated dose of vitamins, minerals and antioxidants. Juicing does not replace eating food, but it's a great addition to your Joyous Detox.

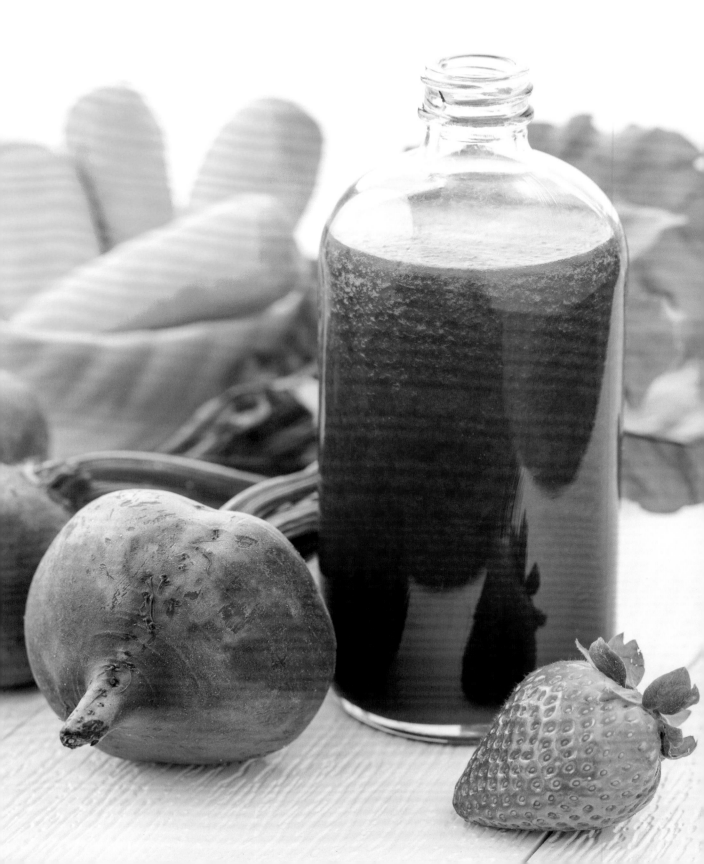

Beet and Strawberry Detox Juice

Beets have an earthy taste, which is softened by the natural sweetness of the strawberries—the two are a perfect combination! This is great on an empty stomach before starting the day.

Makes 1 serving

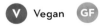 Vegan   Gluten-free   Dairy-free   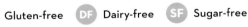 Sugar-free

5 or 6 strawberries

1 medium beet

2 carrots

4 romaine lettuce leaves

Wash all ingredients. Cut vegetables into small chunks that will fit the mouth of your juice extractor. You may add ¼ cup (60 mL) water to the juice extractor at the end to get every last drop of juice. Enjoy immediately.

> ### *Joyous Tip*
> • • •
> Not sure what kind of juicer to use?
> Check out my recommendations on
> page 73. If you want to make any
> of these juices but don't have a juicer,
> whiz everything up in your blender
> and then strain out the pulp.
> For a step-by-step video of this recipe,
> visit my YouTube channel, joyoushealth1.

Green Sparkle Juice

Just like the Green Sparkle Smoothie on page 139, this will help your insides sparkle so your outside glows!

Makes 1 serving

 Vegan   Gluten-free   Dairy-free   Sugar-free

1 apple

4 kale leaves or romaine lettuce leaves

¼ cucumber

¾ cup (175 mL) fresh or frozen pineapple chunks

1 thumb-size piece fresh ginger

Wash all ingredients. Cut fruits and vegetables into small chunks that will fit the mouth of your juice extractor. Remove the seeds from the apple. You may add ¼ cup (60 mL) water to the juice extractor at the end to get every last drop of juice. Enjoy immediately.

Basil Lime Juice

This all-green juice is super tasty and thirst quenching. My favourite time of year to make it is when basil is in season at my local farmers' market. It smells incredible!

Makes 1 serving

 Vegan   Gluten-free   Dairy-free   Sugar-free

1 lime

½ cucumber

2 celery stalks

½ cup (125 mL) chopped fresh basil

Wash all ingredients. Cut lime and vegetables into small chunks that will fit the mouth of your juice extractor. You may add ¼ cup (60 mL) water to the juice extractor at the end to get every last drop of juice. Enjoy immediately.

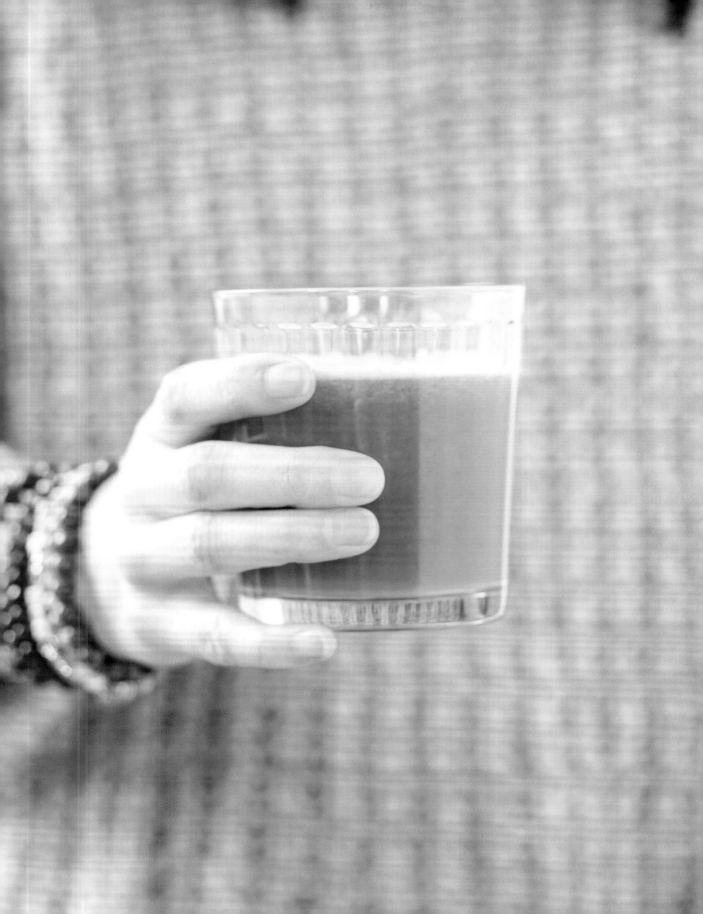

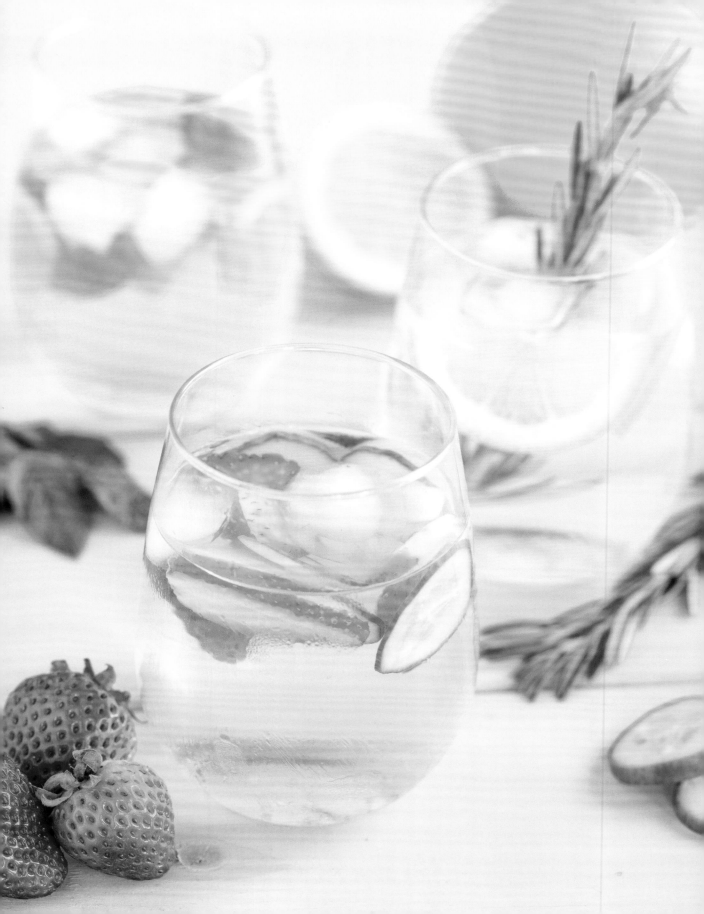

Flavour-Infused Water Three Ways

Most people don't drink enough water, which is essential for detoxification. Here are three ways to add a nice punch of flavour to plain old water—your most inexpensive detox super drink!

Each recipe makes 12 to 16 cups (2.8 to 3.8 L)

 Vegan   **Gluten-free**   **Dairy-free**   **SF** **Sugar-free**

Strawberry Cucumber Basil Water

8 strawberries, halved

3 or 4 fresh basil leaves

1/2 cucumber, sliced crosswise

12 to 16 cups (2.8 to 3.8 L) filtered water

Place strawberries, basil leaves, cucumbers and water in a large jug and refrigerate for at least 2 to 3 hours to let the flavours mingle.

Rosemary Lemon Water

1 to 2 lemons, sliced

2 sprigs fresh rosemary

12 to 16 cups (2.8 to 3.8 L) filtered water

Place lemons, rosemary and water in a large jug and refrigerate for at least 2 to 3 hours to let the flavours mingle.

Orange Mint Water

1 large navel orange, sliced

2 sprigs fresh mint

12 to 16 cups (2.8 to 3.8 L) filtered water

Place oranges, mint and water in a large jug and refrigerate for at least 2 to 3 hours to let the flavours mingle.

Spicy Hot Chocolate

Oh, how I love hot chocolate in the cooler months. This one is kicked up a notch with some spiciness to get your circulation and detox engines going.

Makes 4 to 6 servings

 Vegan Gluten-free Dairy-free Refined Sugar-free

4 cups (1 L) unsweetened almond milk or rice milk

¼ cup (60 mL) raw cacao powder

2 tbsp (30 mL) real maple syrup

1 tsp (5 mL) cinnamon

Pinch of cayenne pepper

In a saucepan, slowly heat almond milk over low heat. When warm, add remaining ingredients. Remove from the heat and blend with an immersion blender until fully combined (or process in a blender). Enjoy right away.

> ## *Joyous Tip*
> • • •
> For a step-by-step video of this recipe, visit my YouTube channel, joyoushealth1.

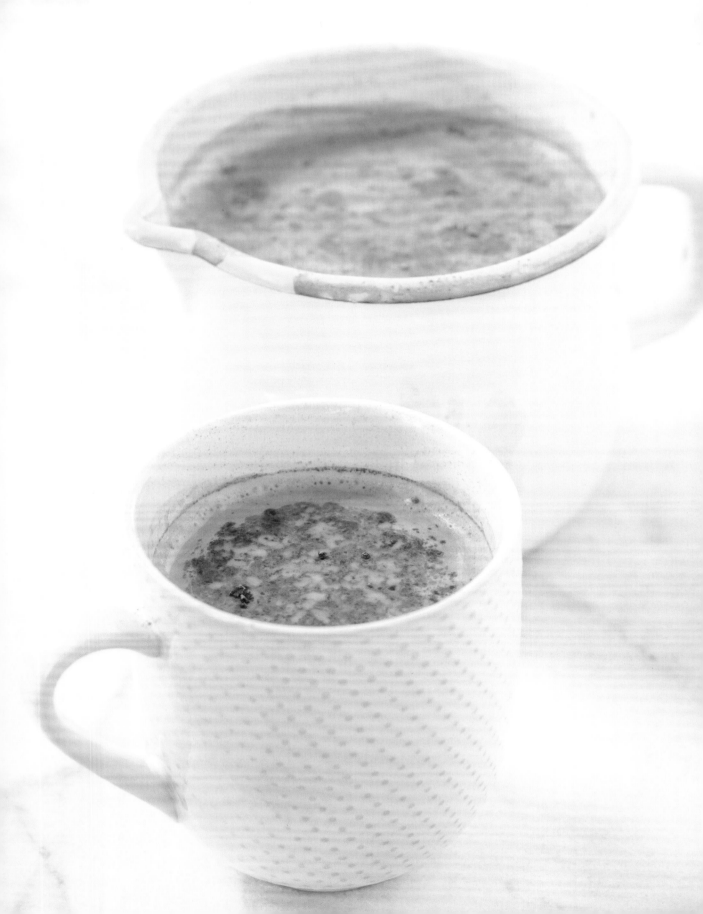

Matcha Coconut Milk Latte

This matcha latte is perfect for a lazy Sunday afternoon and even better if you enjoy it with the No-Bake Carrot Cake Squares with Lemon Icing on page 256.

Makes 1 serving

 Vegetarian   Gluten-free   Dairy-free   Refined Sugar-free

1 tsp (5 mL) matcha green tea powder

¼ cup (60 mL) boiling water

1 cup (250 mL) coconut milk

1 tsp (5 mL) liquid honey

Place matcha powder in a bowl. Add boiling water and whisk until frothy.

Warm coconut milk with a milk frother or in a small pot over very low heat. Pour into a mug and stir in matcha and honey.

> *Joyous Tip*
>
> • • •
>
> Matcha powder can be purchased at a specialty tea shop and most health food stores. Be sure to purchase certified organic matcha, free of pesticides.

Joyous Iced Tea

All throughout the summer I keep tea brewed with fresh fruit in my fridge in a large mason jar. It is both refreshing and rejuvenating, plus it makes hydrating much more tasty! Enjoy this tea with an Energy Booster Ball on page 181.

Makes 10 cups (2.5 L)

 Vegan   Gluten-free   Dairy-free   Sugar-free

3 tbsp (45 mL) your favourite loose-leaf tea

2 cups (500 mL) boiling water

8 cups (2 L) filtered water

Ice

5 strawberries, sliced

Add tea to boiling water. Let steep for 5 minutes. Strain and transfer brewed tea to an extra-large jug or mason jar. Add 8 cups (2 L) water, ice and sliced strawberries. Refrigerate.

Sweet Potato Coconut Soup

The natural sweetness of sweet potatoes in this soup will satisfy your taste buds, and the good fats in the coconut milk will fill up your belly. It is the perfect combination of healthy and tasty in one bowl!

Makes 4 servings

 Vegan Gluten-free Dairy-free Sugar-free

1 tbsp (15 mL) grapeseed oil

2 to 3 shallots, finely chopped

2 garlic cloves, finely chopped

1 cup (250 mL) cooked navy beans

1 cup (250 mL) chopped roasted sweet potatoes

2 cups (500 mL) coconut milk

1/2 cup (125 mL) filtered water

Juice of 1 lemon

Sea salt and pepper

In a medium saucepan, heat grapeseed oil over medium heat. Add shallots and garlic and cook, stirring occasionally, until tender.

Transfer mixture to a high-speed blender or food processor. Add navy beans, sweet potatoes, coconut milk and water. Blend for about 20 seconds so that the soup remains chunky in texture.

Transfer blended soup to a large pot. Season with lemon juice, sea salt and pepper. Reheat but do not let boil. Enjoy immediately.

> *Joyous Tip*
> • • •
> Want to make a larger batch of
> soup? Simply double or triple the
> ingredients. This soup freezes well.

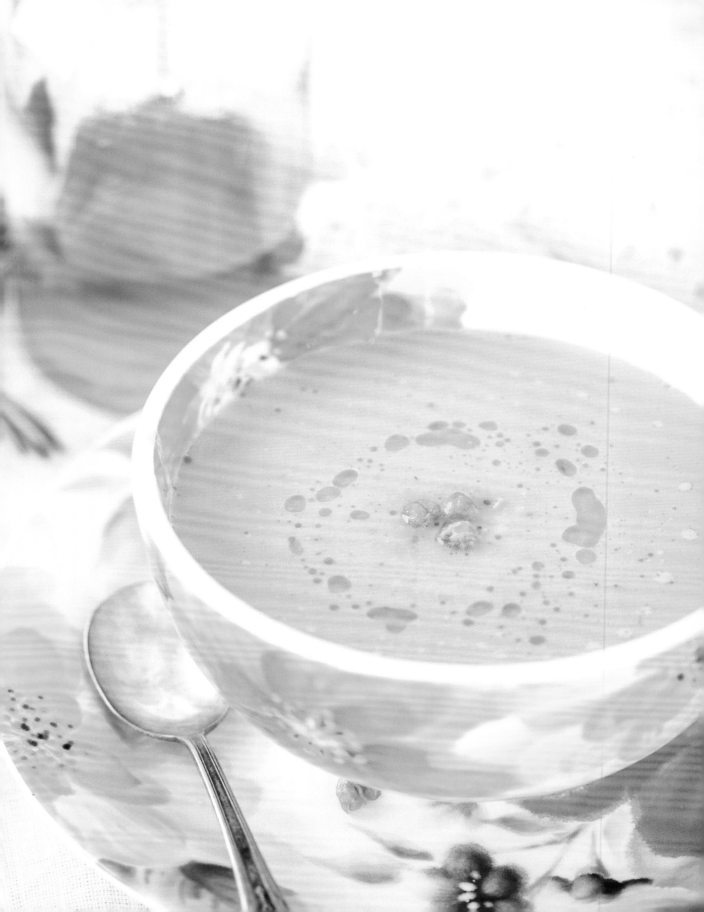

Chickpea Blender Soup

I created this recipe for a segment on the TV show *Steven and Chris*, and it was such a hit it became a regular in my kitchen. The chickpeas give it a great punch of protein, which keeps your detox engine running. I love topping it with the Sea Salt Rosemary Roasted Chickpeas on page 173. For a complete meal, just add a salad.

Makes 6 to 8 servings

 Vegan   Gluten-free   Dairy-free   Sugar-free

2 tbsp (30 mL) grapeseed or coconut oil

1 onion, chopped

1 carrot, chopped

1 celery stalk, chopped

2 cups (500 mL) cooked chickpeas

2 garlic cloves, peeled

2 green onions

½ cup (125 mL) fresh parsley leaves

1½ tsp (7 mL) dried Italian herbs

4 to 6 cups (1 to 1.5 L) vegetable stock

Zest and juice of 1 lemon

Sea salt and pepper

1 tbsp (15 mL) extra-virgin olive oil

In a large pot, heat grapeseed oil over medium heat. Add onions, carrots and celery; cook, stirring occasionally, for 10 minutes or until tender.

Transfer vegetables to a food processor or blender. Add chickpeas, garlic, green onions, parsley, dried herbs, 4 cups (1 L) of the vegetable stock, and lemon zest and juice. Process until smooth. Add more vegetable stock if you prefer a thinner soup.

Return puréed soup to the pot and reheat. Season with sea salt and pepper. Serve drizzled with extra-virgin olive oil.

Joyous Tip

• • •

Sometimes I like adding organic curry powder for a change.
I suggest 2 tbsp (30 mL). The spices that make up curry
powder are detoxifying and anti-inflammatory.
If you are purchasing canned chickpeas, make sure you
choose BPA-free and look for "no salt added" on the label.

Chicken Quinoa Stew

This super-quick stew doesn't require a crockpot or much waiting time—and believe me, you won't want to wait, because it's deliciously comforting. Of course the longer you let it simmer, the more the flavours mingle and the bigger the taste will be.

Makes 4 to 6 servings

 Gluten-free   Dairy-free   Sugar-free

1½ cans (28 oz/796 mL each) whole tomatoes

¾ cup (175 mL) white quinoa

¾ cup (175 mL) finely chopped carrots

½ cup (125 mL) finely chopped celery

2 garlic cloves, finely chopped

4 cups (1 L) filtered water or chicken stock

2 cups (500 mL) chopped or shredded cooked chicken or turkey (preferably organic)

1 tsp (5 mL) dried Italian herbs

Sea salt and pepper

In a large pot, combine tomatoes, quinoa, carrots, celery, garlic and water. Bring to a gentle boil, then simmer until the quinoa is fully cooked, 15 to 20 minutes. Stir in cooked chicken and dried herbs. Season with sea salt and pepper.

Joyous Tip

• • •

To make things easier, purchase a roasted organic chicken and just tear off bite-size pieces.
If you're not using "pre-washed" quinoa, be sure to give it
a good rinse under water before cooking.
If you prefer a thinner consistency, add another 1 cup (250 mL) water or stock.
You can sauté the celery, carrot and garlic first, but I've skipped this step. Not only
is it a time-saver, but you maintain more of the rich minerals in the vegetables if
everything cooks together, rather than sautéing ahead of time.

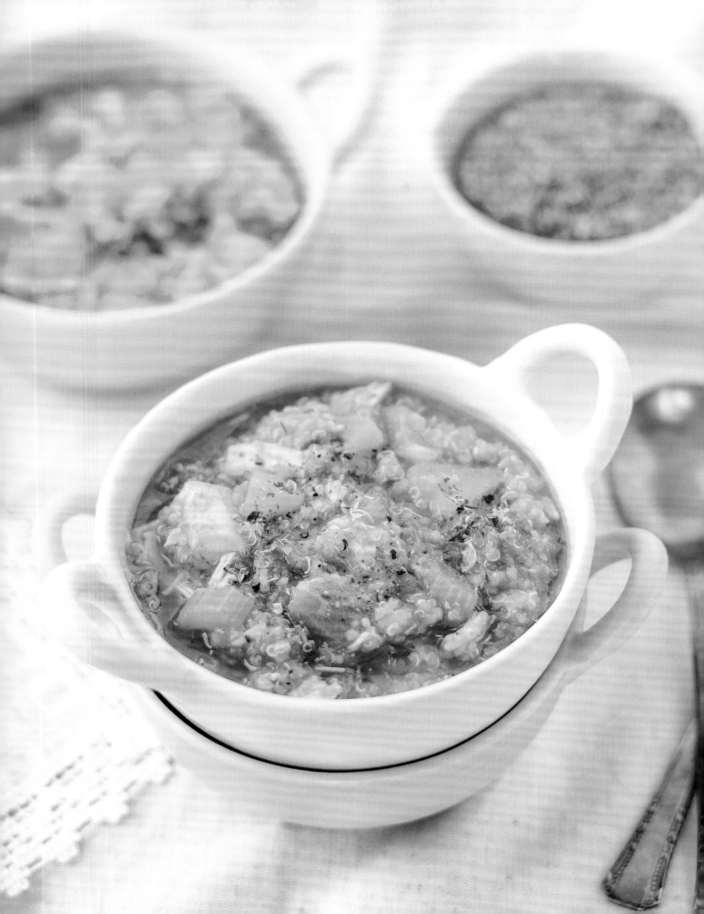

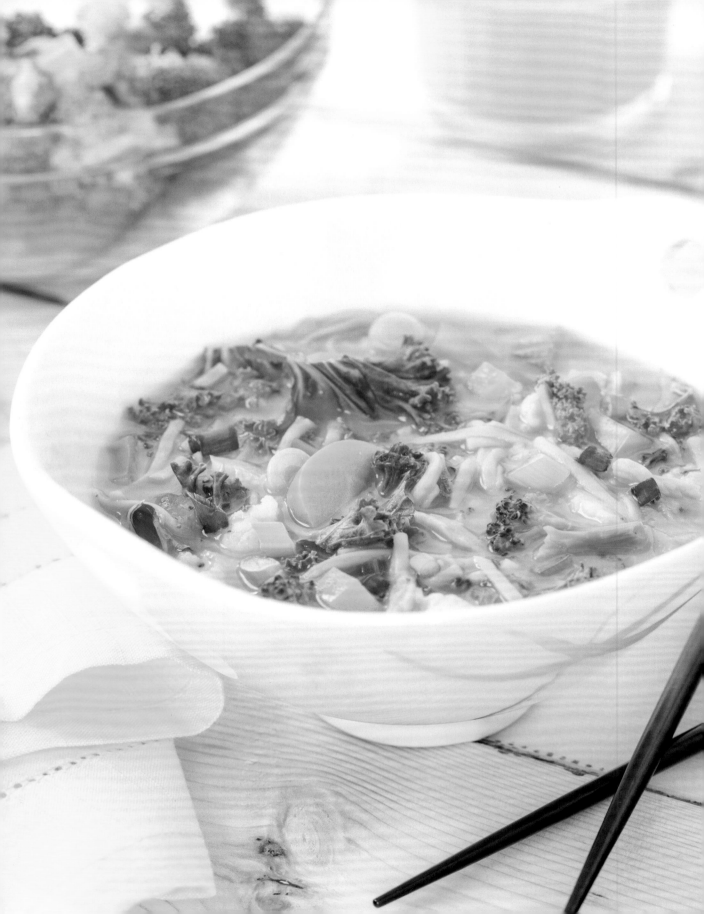

Miso Vegetable Soup

This soup can be enjoyed any time of year because it's nice and light.

Makes 4 servings

 Gluten-free   **Dairy-free**   **Sugar-free**

6 cups (1.5 L) chicken or vegetable stock

2 to 3 tbsp (30 to 45 mL) miso paste

2 carrots, finely chopped

2 celery stalks, finely chopped

2 to 3 garlic cloves, minced

1 cup (250 mL) chopped cauliflower

1 cup (250 mL) chopped broccoli

4 oz (115 g) buckwheat noodles

4 kale leaves, centre stems removed, chopped

2 tbsp (30 mL) gluten-free tamari sauce

Garnishes

2 green onions, thinly sliced

1 tbsp (15 mL) chopped fresh cilantro

Hot sauce (optional)

In a large pot, bring the stock to a gentle boil. In a small bowl, stir together miso paste and a few tablespoons (30 mL) of the simmering stock, then return miso mixture to the pot.

Add carrots, celery, garlic, cauliflower and broccoli. Reduce heat and simmer for 12 minutes. Add noodles, kale and tamari sauce. Simmer until noodles are soft, 5 to 8 minutes. Pour soup into bowls and garnish with green onions, cilantro and hot sauce if using. Enjoy immediately,

Joyous Tip

• • •

Buckwheat noodles have a tendency to clump together. If you want to avoid this, cook them separately as follows:

1. Bring a large pot of water to a boil. Add the noodles and cook according to package instructions.
2. Meanwhile, fill a large bowl with ice-cold water.
3. Drain the cooked noodles. Transfer to the ice water to wash off excess starch.
4. Drain the noodles again and add them to the soup just before serving. Make sure the soup is hot so it warms the noodles.

Miso is a paste made from fermented soybeans. It's fantastic for digestion because it feeds the good bacteria and strengthens the immune system. Look for it at health food stores. Buy certified organic to guarantee it is not made from genetically modified soybeans.

Refreshing Sweet Pea Soup

I absolutely love this soup—the colour, the taste, everything! It reminds me of spring and picking sweet peas from Ma McCarthy's garden. Of course, you can make it any time of year and use frozen peas instead. The flavours are super refreshing and delightful.

Makes 4 servings

 Vegan   Gluten-free   Dairy-free   Sugar-free

1 tbsp (15 mL) extra-virgin olive oil

1 bunch green onions, chopped

2 garlic cloves, finely chopped

3 cups (750 mL) filtered water or veggie stock

4 cups (1 L) fresh or frozen green peas

2 tsp (10 mL) dried tarragon

1/4 cup (60 mL) chopped fresh mint

Juice of 1/2 lemon or lime

Sea salt and pepper

Slivered almonds, for garnish

In a large pot over medium heat, heat olive oil diluted with a small amount of water. Add green onions and garlic; cook, stirring frequently, until tender. Add 2 cups (500 mL) of the water and bring to a gentle boil. Add peas, reduce heat and simmer until peas are tender, about 4 minutes. Add tarragon. Remove from heat and add mint and remaining 1 cup (250 mL) water. Season with lemon juice, sea salt and pepper.

Using an immersion blender, purée until smooth (or let cool slightly and purée in a blender). Soup can be served warm or chilled. Pour into bowls and garnish with slivered almonds.

Joyous Tip

• • •

Not only are peas a wonderful food for detoxification because they are a good source of fibre, but they are also a total beauty food to help you glow from the inside out. This is thanks to the beauty trio of nutrients: vitamins A, C and K.

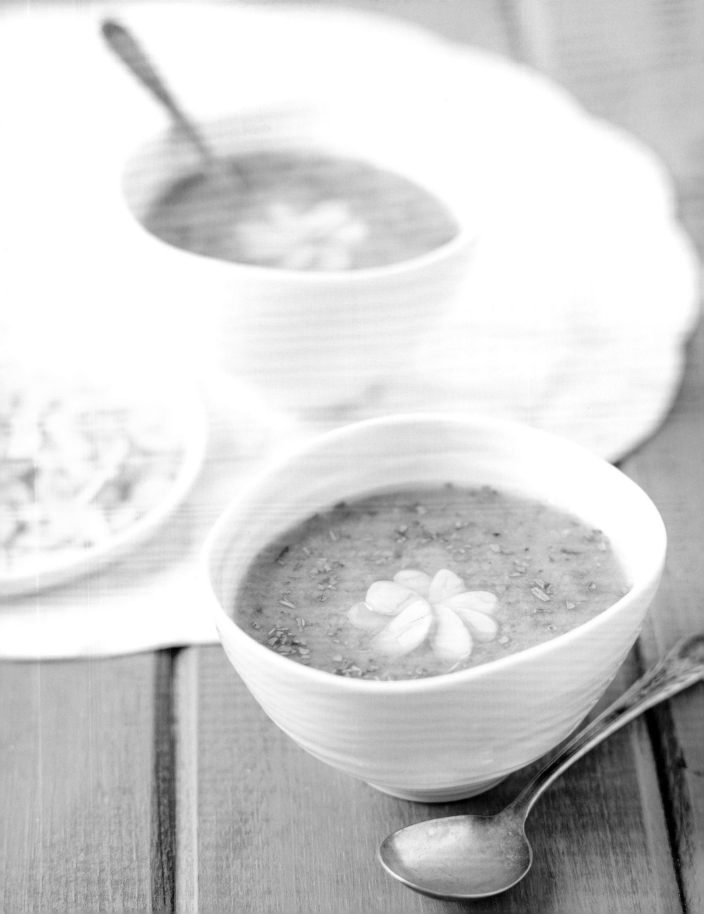

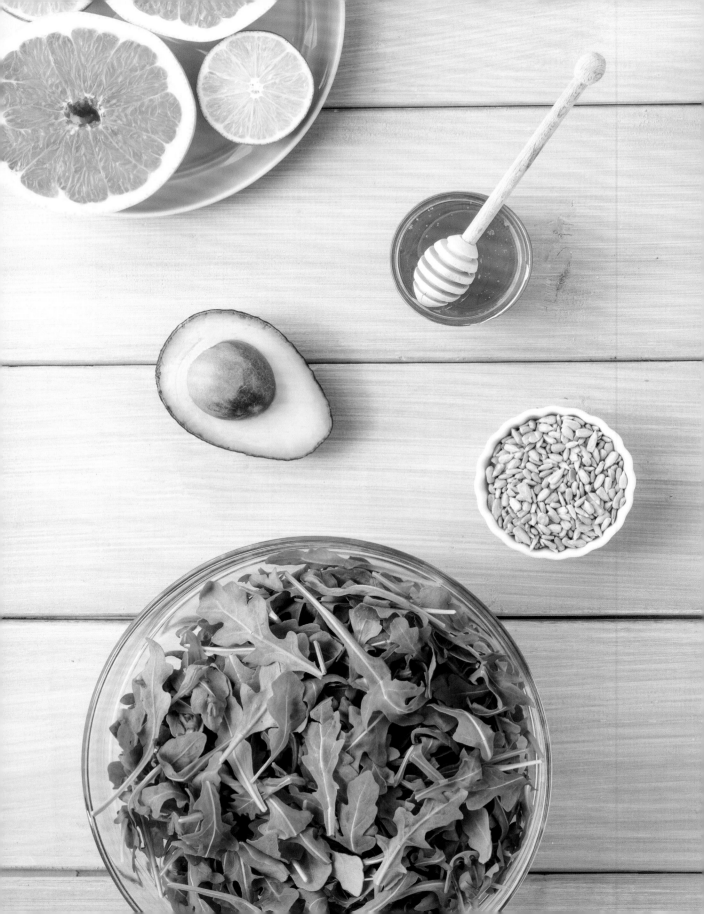

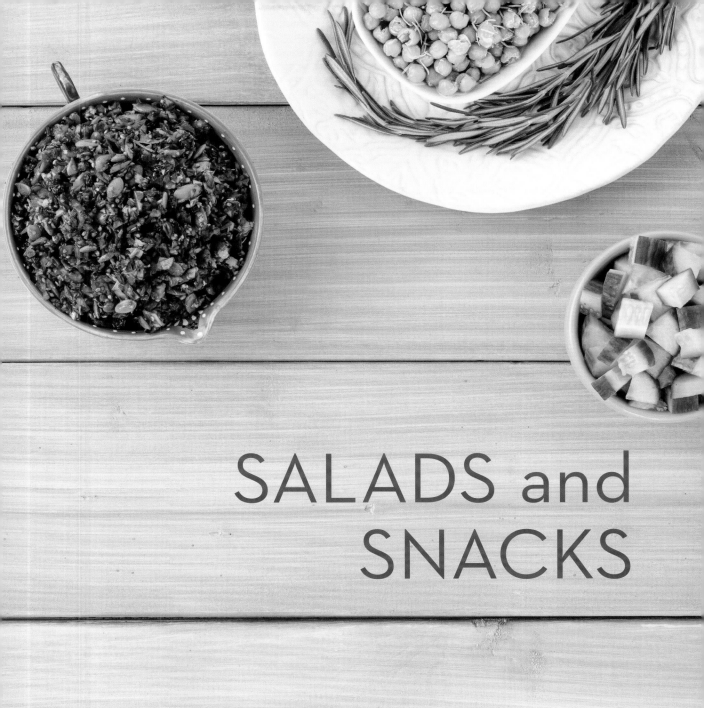

SALADS and SNACKS

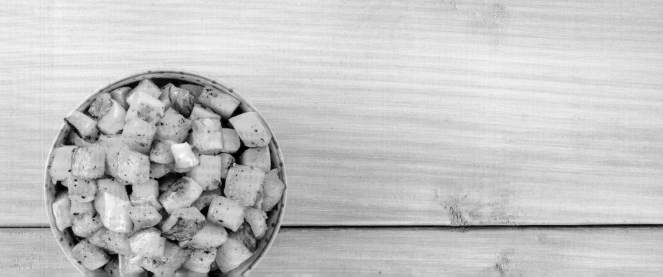

Cinnamon Roasted Chickpeas

Here's a sweet take on roasted chickpeas.

Makes 1¹/₂ cups (375 mL)

 Vegan **Gluten-free** **Dairy-free** RSF **Refined Sugar-free**

1¹/₂ cups (375 mL) cooked chickpeas, dried well

1 tbsp (15 mL) coconut oil, melted

1 tsp (5 mL) coconut sugar or real maple syrup

1 tsp (5 mL) cinnamon

Preheat oven to 375°F (190°C). Line a baking sheet with parchment paper.

In a medium bowl, toss together chickpeas, coconut oil, coconut sugar and cinnamon until well coated. Spread chickpeas on the baking sheet. Bake for 30 minutes or until crisp.

Spicy Roasted Chickpeas

Kick things up a notch taste-wise while you give your metabolism a boost with these spicy chickpeas.

Makes 1¹/₂ cups (375 mL)

 Vegan **Gluten-free** **Dairy-free** **Sugar-free**

1¹/₂ cups (375 mL) cooked chickpeas,
    dried well

1 tbsp (15 mL) grapeseed oil

1 tsp (5 mL) turmeric

¹/₂ tsp (2 mL) cayenne pepper

¹/₂ tsp (2 mL) fine sea salt

Preheat oven to 375°F (190°C). Line a baking sheet with parchment paper.

In a medium bowl, toss together chickpeas, grapeseed oil, turmeric, cayenne and sea salt until well coated. Spread chickpeas on the baking sheet. Bake for 30 minutes or until crisp.

> *Joyous Tip*
>
> • • •
>
> Whether you're using home-cooked or canned chickpeas, be sure to dry them really well. This will help the oil, coconut sugar and cinnamon stick better.

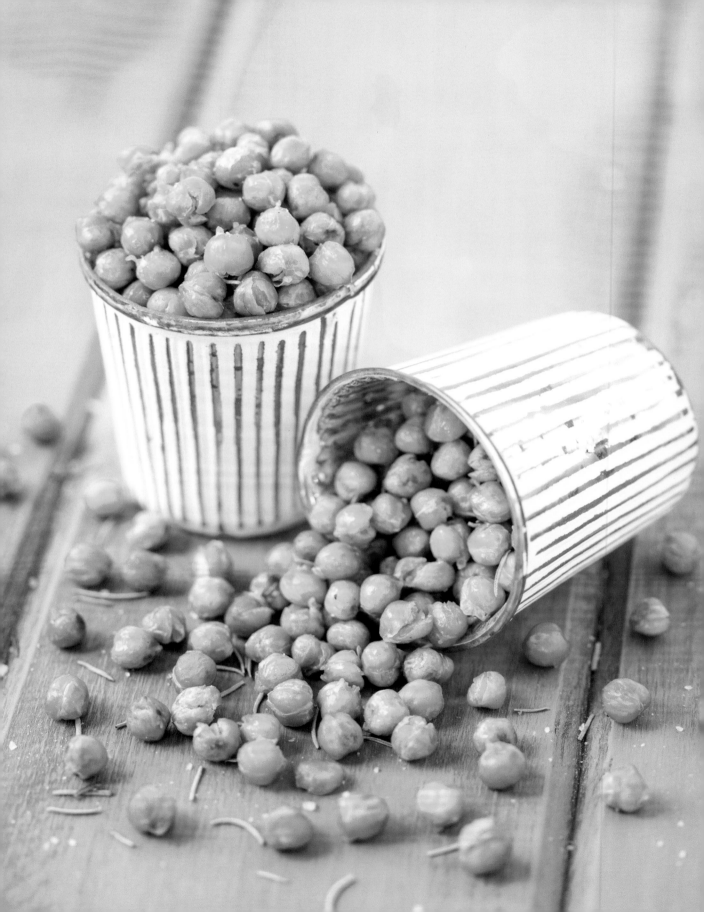

Sea Salt Rosemary Roasted Chickpeas

These crunchy salty bites of deliciousness totally kill a chip craving. Plus, they have protein and tons of fibre and minerals, unlike junk food snacks!

Makes 1¹/₂ cups (375 mL)

 Vegan   **Gluten-free**   **Dairy-free**   **Sugar-free**

1¹/₂ cups (375 mL) cooked chickpeas, dried well

1 tbsp (15 mL) grapeseed oil

1 tsp (5 mL) dried rosemary

¹/₂ tsp (2 mL) fine sea salt

Preheat oven to 375°F (190°C). Line a baking sheet with parchment paper.

In a medium bowl, toss together chickpeas, grapeseed oil, rosemary and sea salt until well coated. Spread chickpeas on the baking sheet. Bake for 30 minutes or until crisp.

> ## Joyous Tip
> • • •
>
> Be sure to dry the chickpeas really well. This will help the oil and seasonings stick better.
> Chickpeas are incredible for your digestive and detoxification systems. They are a rich source of insoluble fibre, which remains undigested until it reaches the last part of your large intestine. Here it becomes a valuable fuel source for the bacteria in your colon, which produce short-chain fatty acids that feed the cells of your intestinal wall. This can help reduce the risk of certain cancers, including colon cancer. Plus, this same fibre helps to control your appetite.

Cinnamon Pecan Butter

This is my favourite nut butter. The good fats, fibre and protein fill you up, making this nut butter a great way to keep hunger at bay. For a mid-afternoon pick-me-up, slice up some apples and slather on some of this butter.

Makes approximately 2 cups (500 mL)

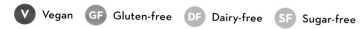 **Vegan** **GF** **Gluten-free** **DF** **Dairy-free** **SF** **Sugar-free**

2 cups (500 mL) whole raw pecans

2 tsp (10 mL) cinnamon

Pinch of sea salt

Preheat oven to 300°F (150°C). Line a baking sheet with parchment paper.

Spread pecans evenly on baking sheet and bake for 10 to 12 minutes, until fragrant. Be careful not to burn them.

Transfer pecans to a food processor or blender and add cinnamon and sea salt. Pulse until creamy smooth. Transfer to a glass jar with a tight-fitting lid and store in the fridge for up to 2 weeks.

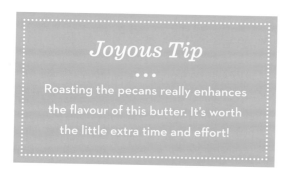

Joyous Tip

• • •

Roasting the pecans really enhances the flavour of this butter. It's worth the little extra time and effort!

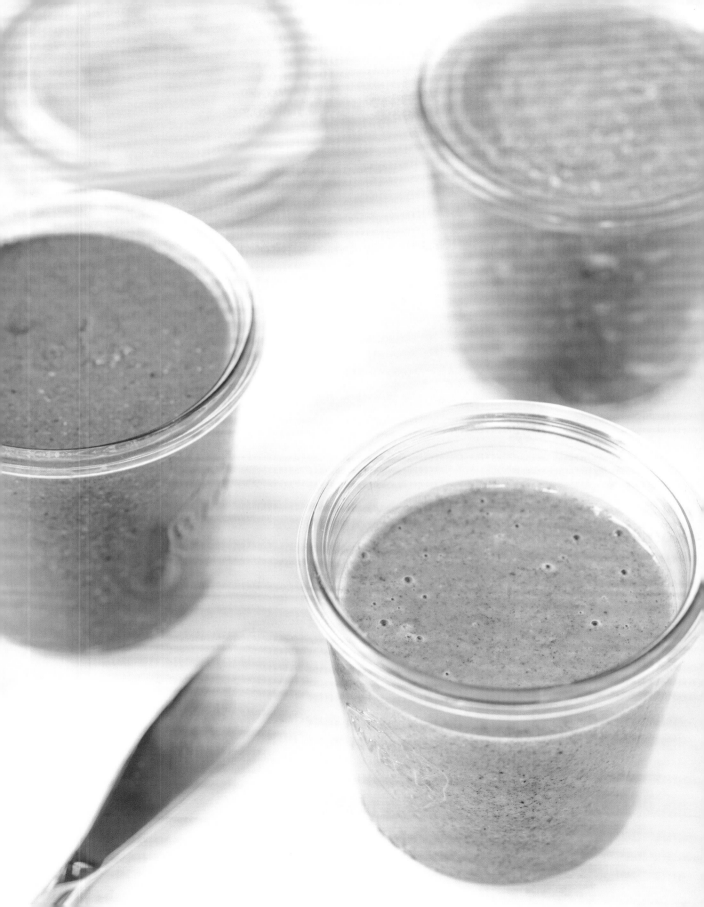

Chocolate Almond Butter

Almonds are a wonderful source of magnesium and vitamin E. They have more protein per ounce than any other tree nut. The raw cacao turns this butter into a guilt-free chocolate treat.

Makes approximately 2 cups (500 mL)

 Vegan   Gluten-free   Dairy-free   Refined Sugar-free

2 cups (500 mL) whole raw almonds

3 tbsp (45 mL) raw cacao powder

Pinch of sea salt

2 to 4 tbsp (30 to 60 mL) dark real maple syrup (optional)

Preheat oven to 300°F (150°C). Line a baking sheet with parchment paper.

Spread almonds evenly on baking sheet and bake for 10 to 12 minutes, until fragrant. Be careful not to burn them.

Transfer almonds to a food processor or blender and add cacao powder and sea salt. Pulse until creamy smooth. Add 2 tbsp (30 mL) maple syrup, if using. If you want it a touch sweeter, add more maple syrup and pulse again. Transfer to a glass jar with a tight lid and store in the fridge for up to 2 weeks.

> *Joyous Tip*
>
> • • •
>
> You can also make this nut butter without roasting the almonds if you want a raw version of the recipe.

Sunflower and Hemp Honey Orange Butter

Seeds are a wonderful nutrient-rich alternative to nut butters. I absolutely love the flavour of the orange in this recipe. Enjoy on toast, on crackers or on sliced fruit.

Makes approximately 2 cups (500 mL)

 Vegetarian Gluten-free Dairy-free Refined Sugar-free

1 cup (250 mL) raw sunflower seeds

1 cup (250 mL) shelled hemp seeds

¼ cup (60 mL) liquid honey

Zest of 1 organic orange

Soak sunflower seeds in water to cover for 4 hours. Drain.

Place all ingredients in a blender or food processor and blend until smooth. Transfer to a glass jar with a tight-fitting lid and store in the fridge for up to 1 week.

> ## *Joyous Tip*
> • • •
> Sunflower seeds are a good source of nutrients that protect the body during a detox and enhance detoxification systems, among them vitamin E; B vitamins including folate, B_1 and B_6; and magnesium and selenium.

Blueberry Chia Jam

Once you start making your own chia jam, you'll never buy that sugar-filled store-bought jam again. The chia seeds make this jam fantastic for digestion and elimination. Enjoy with the Best Ever Cinnamon Flaxseed Bread on page 127.

Makes approximately 1 cup (250 mL)

 Vegan   Gluten-free   Dairy-free   Sugar-free

1¼ cups (300 mL) fresh or thawed frozen wild blueberries
1 tbsp (15 mL) chia seeds
½ tsp (2 mL) pure vanilla extract

Place all ingredients in a food processor and blend until smooth. Transfer to an airtight container and refrigerate overnight before using. Jam keeps for 7 to 10 days in the fridge.

Apple Cinnamon Chia Jam

This jam smells and tastes like apple pie. Many recipes don't call for enough cinnamon in my opinion, so you'll get a mega-dose of this detox superfood in this recipe!

Makes approximately 1 cup (250 mL)

 Vegan   Gluten-free   Dairy-free   Sugar-free

2 large apples (unpeeled if organic), cored and cut into chunks
1 tbsp (15 mL) chia seeds
1 tbsp (15 mL) cinnamon
½ tsp (2 mL) pure vanilla extract

Place all ingredients in a food processor and blend until smooth. Transfer to an airtight container and refrigerate overnight before using. Jam keeps for 7 to 10 days in the fridge.

> ## Joyous Tip
> • • •
> Chia is a detox superfood. Because of its high fibre content it helps to absorb toxins from the digestive system. It also aids in balancing the blood sugar, which keeps those cravings in check!

Peach Coconut Chia Jam

My favourite time of year to make this jam is when peaches are in season. You'll love the addition of the coconut butter for fibre, good fat, protein and taste.

Makes approximately 1 cup (250 mL)

 Vegan Gluten-free Dairy-free Sugar-free

2 to 3 medium peaches (unpeeled), pitted and cut into chunks

1 tbsp (15 mL) chia seeds

1 tbsp (15 mL) unsweetened, unsulphured shredded coconut

1 tbsp (15 mL) coconut butter

Place all ingredients in a food processor and blend until smooth. Transfer to an airtight container and refrigerate overnight before using. Jam keeps for 7 to 10 days in the fridge.

> *Joyous Tip*
>
> • • •
>
> Note that this recipe uses coconut butter, not coconut oil. Coconut butter is made from the whole flesh of the coconut. It includes the good fat (oil), fibre and protein. It is sweeter than coconut oil but just as health-promoting.

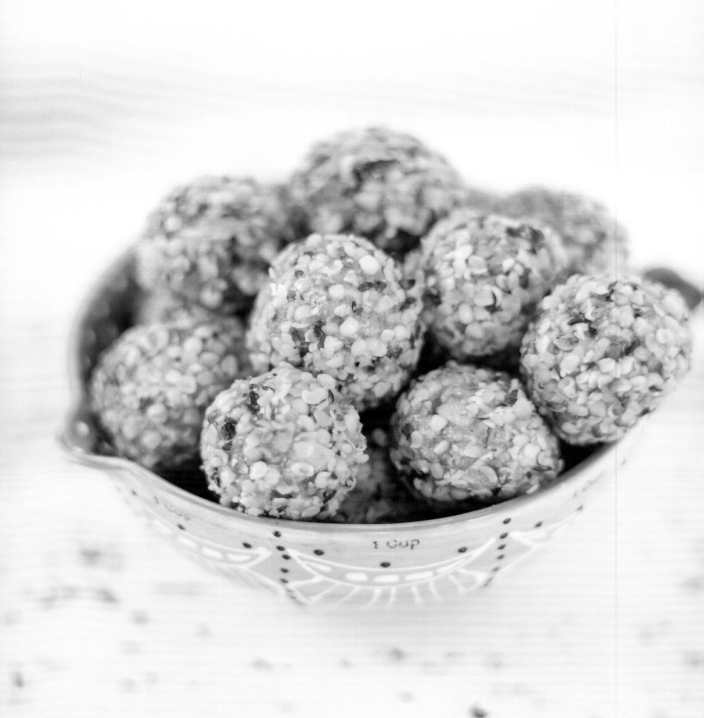

Energy Booster Balls

I keep these handy in my freezer for when I need a quick energy boost, especially on days when I'm strapped for time to keep me on track health-wise. They are super tasty and will tide you over between meals.

Makes 18 to 24 balls

 Vegetarian   **Gluten-free**   **Dairy-free**   **Refined Sugar-free**

2 cups (500 mL) Grain-Free Nutty Granola (page 114)
½ cup (125 mL) almond butter
¼ cup (60 mL) liquid honey
½ cup (125 mL) shelled hemp seeds

Pulse granola in a food processor to a slightly finer texture, but not a powder (this will make it easier to form into balls). Transfer to a large bowl and add almond butter and honey. Mix well, then roll into 1-inch (2.5 cm) balls.

Place the hemp seeds in a small bowl. Roll each ball in the hemp seeds to coat evenly. Arrange balls on a parchment-lined baking sheet and freeze until firm, at least 4 hours. Keep frozen.

> ## *Joyous Tip*
> • • •
> Want to make them nut-free? Swap the almond butter for sunflower or pumpkin seed butter. They are just as delicious! Almonds are a detox superfood. They make the perfect nut butter for this recipe because the good fat and protein really help to smash carb cravings.

Hemp Heart Spinach Spread

Forget the mayo-heavy spinach dip inside the pumpernickel bread that was so popular a few decades back. This healthy version of spinach dip has more flavour and is a nutrition powerhouse full of detoxifying fibre and protein to keep you satisfied. Serve with crisp gluten-free crackers or chopped crunchy veggies.

Makes 1 to 1 1/2 cups (250 to 375 mL)

 Vegan   Gluten-free   Dairy-free   Sugar-free

2 cups (500 mL) loosely packed fresh spinach, washed

1 to 2 garlic cloves, peeled

1/3 cup (75 mL) shelled hemp seeds

1/3 cup (75 mL) drained oil-packed sun-dried tomatoes

2 tbsp (30 mL) lemon juice

1/2 tsp (2 mL) sea salt

1/4 tsp (1 mL) cayenne pepper

Place all ingredients in a food processor or blender. Blend until desired consistency, either smooth or with some soft chunks. Store in an airtight container in the fridge for up to 1 week.

> ## *Joyous Tip*
> • • •
> Spinach is a source of nutrients that increase an important detox compound called alpha-lipoic acid. Anything green is a rich source of chlorophyll that encourages detox of environmental chemicals.

Chopped Kale and Beet Salad

Kale and beets together make the ultimate detox salad. I love making this salad after I've picked up the ingredients at my local farmers' market.

Makes 6 servings

 Vegetarian Gluten-free Dairy-free **RSF** Refined Sugar-free

Salad

2 bunches kale, centre stems removed, finely
    chopped
4 medium beets (unpeeled if organic), grated
    (2 cups/500 mL)
1/3 cup (75 mL) pumpkin seeds
6 Medjool dates, pitted and chopped

Dressing

Juice of 1 lemon
1/3 cup (75 mL) extra-virgin olive oil
2 tbsp (30 mL) liquid honey
1/2 tsp (2 mL) sea salt

In a large salad bowl, combine kale, beets, pumpkin seeds and dates. Whisk dressing ingredients together in a small bowl. Pour over salad and toss.

> *Joyous Tip*
> • • •
> The secret to a great kale salad is to finely chop the kale. Chopping breaks down kale's tough fibres, making it easier to chew and digest.

Citrus Fennel Salad with Toasted Sunflower Seeds

This gorgeous salad doesn't need an introduction—just the photo makes my mouth water. The combination of bright flavours will delight your taste buds and cleanse your body.

Makes 6 to 8 servings

 Vegetarian   Gluten-free   Dairy-free   Refined Sugar-free

Toasted Sunflower Seeds

1 cup (250 mL) raw sunflower or pumpkin seeds

1 tbsp (15 mL) grapeseed oil

¼ tsp (1 mL) cinnamon

¼ tsp (1 mL) nutmeg

⅛ tsp (0.5 mL) ground cloves

Pinch of fine sea salt

Salad

2 grapefruit (pink or red)

2 large oranges

2 fennel bulbs, trimmed, halved, cored and thinly sliced on a mandoline

2 tbsp (30 mL) finely chopped fresh mint

2 tbsp (30 mL) extra-virgin olive oil

1 tbsp (15 mL) liquid honey

Juice of ½ lemon

Juice of ¼ grapefruit

Pinch of sea salt

Preheat oven to 350°F (180°C).

To make the toasted sunflower seeds, in a large bowl, combine all ingredients. Mix to coat well. Spread evenly on a parchment-lined baking sheet and lightly toast in the oven for 5 to 7 minutes or until lightly golden. Watch carefully so they don't burn. Remove from oven and set aside.

To make the salad, peel grapefruit and oranges. (You may wish to remove the white pith from the citrus, but it's not necessary and contains vitamin C.) Cut the fruit segments into small triangular chunks and transfer to a large bowl. Add fennel and mint.

In a small bowl, whisk together olive oil, honey, lemon juice and grapefruit juice. Pour dressing over salad and toss. Top with toasted sunflower seeds and season with sea salt.

> ## Joyous Tip
> • • •
> A rich source of fibre, fennel is a detox superfood.
> It is also very hydrating, making it ideal for digestion.

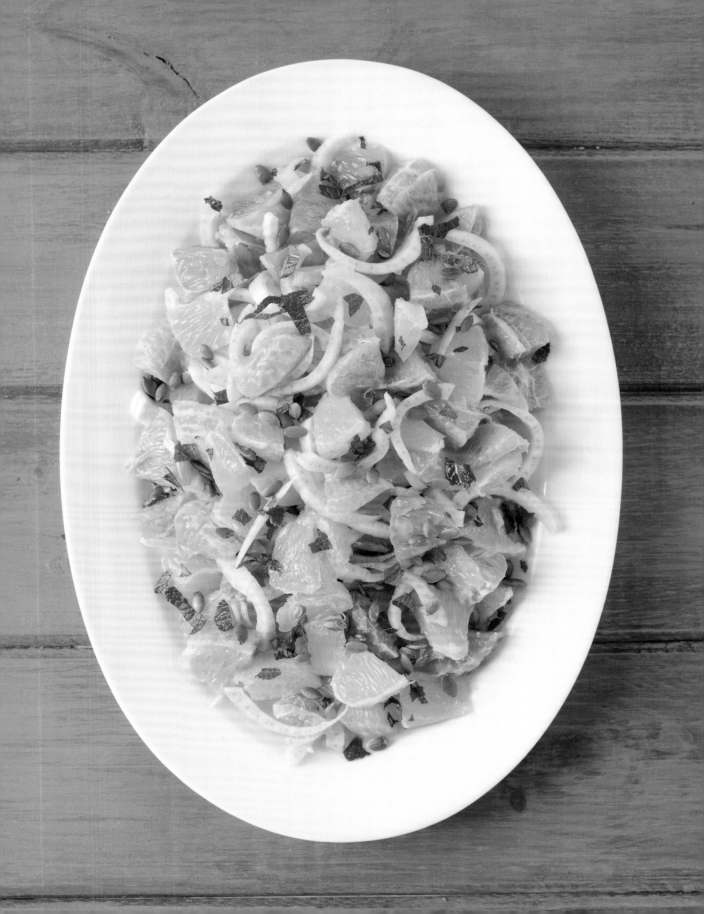

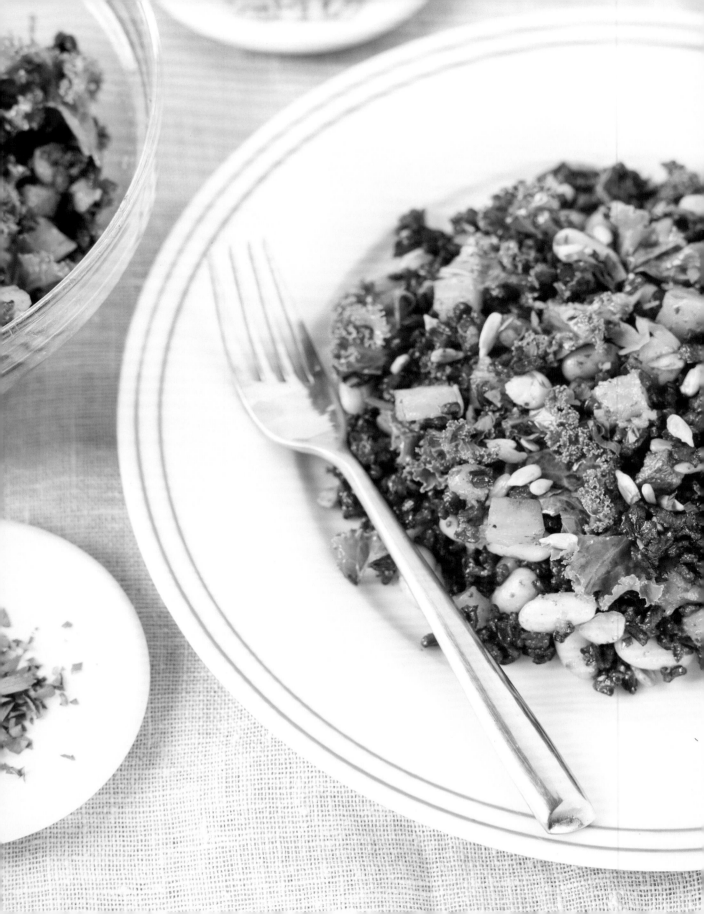

Black Rice Butternut Squash Salad

I don't know about you, but I get bored eating the same grains week after week. Black rice is a welcome change, and it is bursting with nutrients. In fact, it has double the amount of fibre as brown rice. An added bonus is that it's packed with antioxidants too.

Makes 4 to 6 servings

 Vegan Gluten-free Dairy-free Sugar-free

5 to 6 large kale leaves or Swiss chard

½ butternut squash, peeled, seeded and cubed

3 tbsp (45 mL) coconut oil

¼ cup (60 mL) raw sunflower seeds

2 large garlic cloves, crushed

2 tsp (10 mL) curry powder

2 tsp (10 mL) cumin seeds

1 cup (250 mL) cooked navy beans

1½ cups (375 mL) cooked black rice

3 tbsp (45 mL) coarsely chopped fresh parsley

Sea salt and freshly ground black pepper

4 tsp (20 mL) extra-virgin olive oil

Cut away and discard centre stems from kale or Swiss chard, then tear or slice leaves into medium-size pieces. Set aside. You can prepare the butternut squash one of two ways:

1. Bring water to a boil in a medium pot. Add squash and boil for 7 to 15 minutes, until soft but not mushy. Drain, set aside and let cool.

2. Preheat oven to 375°F (190°C). Place butternut squash in a baking dish, drizzle with extra-virgin olive oil, cover and bake for 30 to 35 minutes, until soft but not mushy. Let cool.

Melt coconut oil in a large saucepan over medium heat. Add sunflower seeds and cook for about 2 minutes, stirring constantly until golden brown. Remove sunflower seeds and set aside.

Increase heat to medium-high. Add garlic, curry and cumin seeds; cook, stirring, for 1 minute. Add more coconut oil if needed. Add cooked squash, kale or Swiss chard and navy beans; cook, stirring, for 2 to 4 minutes, until vegetables are heated through.

Transfer mixture to a large bowl. Add black rice, parsley and sunflower seeds. Toss gently to combine. Season with sea salt and pepper. Serve warm, drizzled with extra-virgin olive oil. Keeps in the fridge, in an airtight container, for up to 3 days.

> ## Joyous Tip
> • • •
> Black rice takes about 45 minutes to cook.
> I normally cook it the day before to save time.

Mason Jar Salad Three Ways

Rainbow Mason Jar Salad

Super-portable, mason jars are my go-to for food storage. The colours in this salad remind me of a rainbow. A rainbow of colours from real, whole foods indicates a high level of phytonutrients (plant medicines), many of which aid in detoxification.

Makes 1 serving

 Vegan   Gluten-free   Dairy-free   **SF** Sugar-free

Rainbow Salad

¾ cup (175 mL) cooked white quinoa

2 carrots, grated or chopped

¼ cup (60 mL) finely chopped purple cabbage

⅓ cup (75 mL) chopped cucumber

4 or 5 grape or cherry tomatoes

½ cup (125 mL) arugula or other leafy greens

Sprinkle of finely chopped green onion

Dressing

Juice of ½ lemon

½ garlic clove, finely minced

2 to 3 tbsp (30 to 45 mL) extra-virgin olive oil

¼ tsp (1 mL) dried Italian herbs

To make the salad, layer quinoa in a pint (500 mL) mason jar. Layer remaining salad ingredients in the order listed, with the heaviest at the bottom, building up to the lightest on top.

To make the dressing, whisk together all ingredients in a small bowl.

> *Joyous Tip*
> • • •
> If you will be eating this salad later, put the dressing in a separate container and add it just before eating.

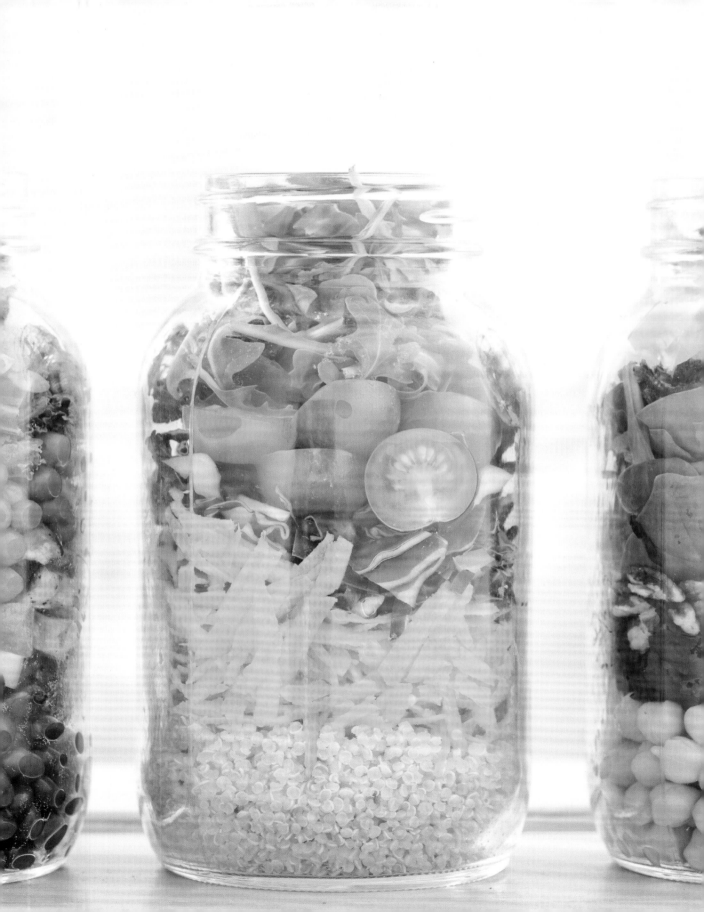

Give Thanks Mason Jar Salad

The ingredients in this salad remind me of Thanksgiving—beets, spinach, cranberries and pecans. This is a wonderful opportunity to be thankful for this nourishing meal!

Makes 1 serving

 Vegetarian   **Gluten-free**   **Dairy-free** **RSF** **Refined Sugar-free**

Give Thanks Salad

½ cup (125 mL) cooked chickpeas

½ medium beet (unpeeled if organic), grated or finely chopped

2 tbsp (30 mL) chopped pecans

½ cup (125 mL) fresh spinach

2 tbsp (30 mL) dried cranberries

½ cup (125 mL) chopped yellow or green sweet pepper

1 tbsp (15 mL) finely chopped red onion

Dressing

2 to 3 tbsp (30 to 45 mL) extra-virgin olive oil

1 tsp (5 mL) apple cider vinegar

1 tsp (5 mL) liquid honey

To make the salad, layer chickpeas in a pint (500 mL) mason jar. Layer remaining salad ingredients in the order listed, with the heaviest at the bottom, building up to the lightest on top.

To make the dressing, whisk together all ingredients in a small bowl.

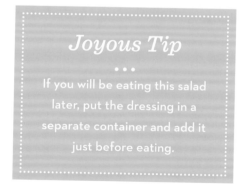

Joyous Tip

• • •

If you will be eating this salad later, put the dressing in a separate container and add it just before eating.

Harvest Mason Jar Salad

I love the fall because farmers' markets are bursting with squash and kale—two amazing detox-friendly foods, rich with fibre.

Makes 1 serving

 Vegan   Gluten-free   Dairy-free   Sugar-free

Harvest Salad

³/₄ cup (375 mL) cooked black beans

¹/₃ cup (75 mL) chopped zucchini

¹/₃ cup (75 mL) chopped cooked sweet potato or butternut squash

¹/₂ cup (125 mL) finely chopped kale (centre stems removed)

¹/₄ cup (60 mL) green peas

4 or 5 broccoli florets

2 tbsp (30 mL) raw pumpkin seeds

Sprinkle of finely chopped green onion

Tahini Lemon Dressing

1 tbsp (15 mL) chopped fresh parsley, cilantro or rosemary

2 tbsp (30 mL) tahini

Juice of 1 lemon

1 tbsp (15 mL) filtered water

To make the salad, layer black beans in a pint (500 mL) mason jar. Add remaining salad ingredients in the order listed, with the heaviest at the bottom, building up to the lightest on top.

To make the dressing, whisk together all ingredients in a small bowl. Add more liquid if you want a thinner consistency.

> *Joyous Tip*
>
> • • •
>
> If you will be eating this salad later, put the dressing in a separate container and add it just before eating.

Everything but the Kitchen Sink Salad with Creamy Dijon Dressing

The name says it all! Need to clean out your fridge? If you've got a great salad dressing like this one, then you have no excuse not to use up all those wonderfully detoxifying veggies.

Makes 6 servings

 Vegan **Gluten-free** **Dairy-free** **Refined Sugar-free**

Creamy Dijon Dressing

1 to 2 garlic cloves, minced

¼ cup (60 mL) lemon juice

¼ cup (60 mL) extra-virgin olive oil

¼ cup (60 mL) tahini

3 tbsp (45 mL) filtered water

1 tbsp (15 mL) Dijon mustard

1 tbsp (15 mL) real maple syrup

Everything Salad

6 cups (1.5 L) mixed greens

3 carrots, chopped

½ cucumber, finely chopped

2 beets (unpeeled if organic), grated

1 sweet pepper, chopped

¼ cup (60 mL) finely chopped red onion

⅓ cup (75 mL) raw pumpkin or sunflower seeds

1 avocado, peeled, pitted and cubed

To make the dressing, whisk all ingredients together in a small bowl. If you want a thinner consistency, add more water or olive oil.

To make the salad, in a large bowl, combine all ingredients except avocado. Toss well. Drizzle with dressing, top with cubed avocado and serve immediately.

Joyous Tip

• • •

Tahini is basically ground sesame seeds. Not only are sesame seeds a rich source of such nutrients as calcium, magnesium, iron, phosphorus, vitamin B₁, zinc and selenium, but they are also a rich source of a special type of fibre called lignans, which have cholesterol-lowering and liver-protective effects. You can find tahini in health food stores or the ethnic foods section of most grocery stores.

Creamy Cashew Veggie Dip

This dip is pretty much guaranteed to make you want to eat more veggies! It has a nice kick to it from the lemon and apple cider vinegar. It's always a crowd-pleaser when I serve it at parties. You'll love it as a salad dressing too.

Makes approximately 2 cups (500 mL)

 Vegan   Gluten-free   Dairy-free   Refined Sugar-free

1½ cups (375 mL) raw cashews

⅓ cup (75 mL) apple cider vinegar

⅓ cup (75 mL) extra-virgin olive oil

3 tbsp (45 mL) lemon juice

2 tbsp (30 mL) real maple syrup or liquid honey

1 tbsp (15 mL) onion powder

2 tsp (10 mL) sea salt

2 garlic cloves, peeled

¼ cup (60 mL) fresh basil leaves

¼ cup (60 mL) fresh parsley leaves

Soak cashews in 1 cup (250 mL) room-temperature water for at least 2 hours. Drain.

Place all ingredients in blender or food processor. Pulse until creamy. Enjoy with crunchy veggie sticks. Dip keeps in the fridge for up to 1 week.

Joyous Tip

• • •

For a step-by-step video of this recipe, visit joyoushealth.com/cashewdip.

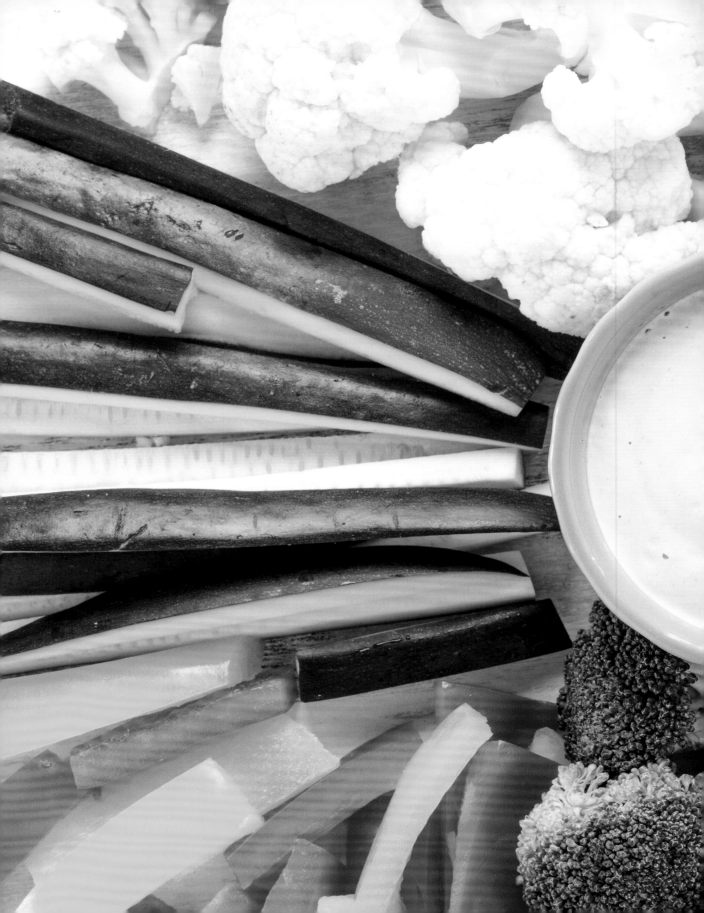

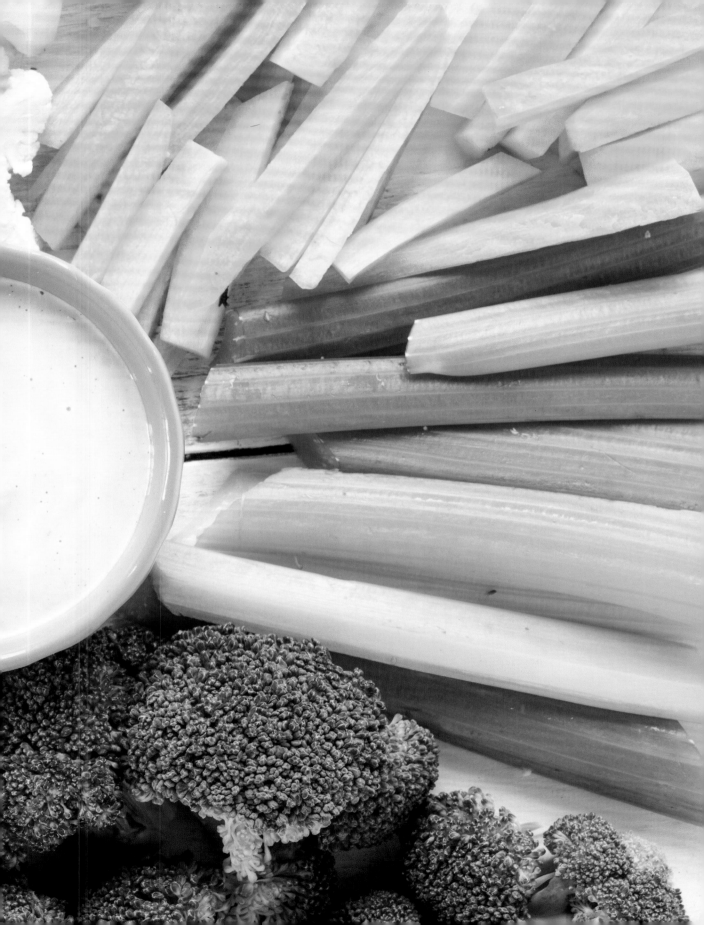

Sun-Dried Tomato Olive Spread

You can never have too many dips and spreads! This one is perfect on gluten-free crackers or, my personal favourite, chopped cucumber. Add a touch more olive oil and enjoy the Sun-Dried Tomato Olive Spread as a dressing for a chilled pasta salad. You could use quinoa, buckwheat or brown rice pasta.

Makes approximately 1 cup (250 mL)

 Vegan   Gluten-free   Dairy-free   Sugar-free

¼ cup (60 mL) raw sunflower seeds

¼ cup (60 mL) raw pumpkin seeds

1 to 2 garlic cloves, peeled

8 oil-packed sun-dried tomatoes, drained

6 olives, pitted

3 to 4 tbsp (45 to 60 mL) extra-virgin olive oil (depending how oily the sun-dried tomatoes are)

Place all ingredients in a food processor. Blend until well combined but not totally smooth. Keeps in the fridge for up to a week.

Almond Arugula Lemon Pesto

The peppery taste of fresh arugula awakens the senses and fires up your detox engines! This pesto is incredibly versatile—enjoy it as a dip, as a pesto for pizza such as the Arugula Pesto Pizza on page 234 or with gluten-free pasta.

Makes approximately 3½ cups (875 mL)

 Vegan   Gluten-free   Dairy-free   Sugar-free

3 cups (750 mL) arugula

½ cup (125 mL) raw almonds

1 garlic clove, peeled

Juice of 1 lemon

2 tbsp (30 mL) extra-virgin olive oil

Sea salt and pepper to taste

Place all ingredients in a food processor or blender. Pulse until desired texture is reached. As a dip, I like it a little chunkier, but for a pesto I blend until it's creamy.

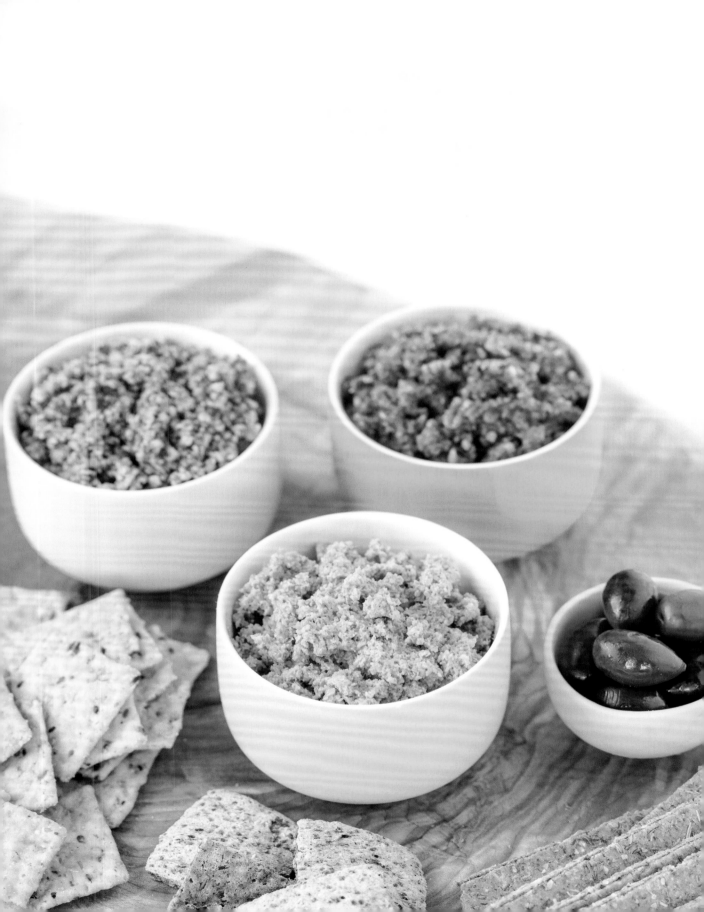

Sunny Punchy Seed Spread

When I first made this spread for a project in a cooking class I was taking, the flavour made me think of sunshine—bright and delicious! It has become my go-to spread when I'm getting tired of ho-hum hummus.

Makes 2 cups (500 mL)

 Vegan   Gluten-free   Dairy-free   Sugar-free

2 cups (500 mL) raw sunflower seeds

2 tsp (10 mL) curry powder

1 garlic clove

¼ cup (60 mL) extra-virgin olive oil

Sea salt and pepper to taste

Soak sunflower seeds in water to cover for 4 hours. Drain.

In a food processor or blender, combine all ingredients. Blend until smooth.

> *Joyous Tip*
>
> • • •
>
> Soaking the seeds releases the enzyme inhibitors, making the seeds much more digestible. It also plumps them up, which is better when making a paste or spread. You can soak any nut or seed and improve their digestibility this way. I don't always soak, but when I'm not whipping something up at the last minute, I will.

Best Ever Hemp Caesar Salad Dressing

This is a variation of the dressing for the Superfood Salad on page 201. Most store-bought creamy Caesar dressings are full of additives like emulsifiers and preservatives—not detox friendly at all.

Makes 1¹/₂ cups (375 mL)

 Vein **Gluten-free** **Dairy-free** **SF** **Sugar-free**

¹/₂ cup (125 mL) raw cashews

¹/₄ cup (60 mL) shelled hemp seeds

1 tsp (5 mL) Dijon mustard

2 garlic cloves, peeled

¹/₂ cup (125 mL) filtered water

¹/₄ cup (60 mL) extra-virgin olive oil

Juice of 1 lemon

Sea salt to taste

Soak cashews in room-temperature water to cover for at least an hour. Drain.

Place all ingredients in a food processor or blender. Blend until smooth. Store in a mason jar in the fridge for 4 to 5 days. Give it a good shake before using.

> *Joyous Tip*
> • • •
> This dressing tastes fabulous
> with chopped raw kale or as
> a dip for raw vegetables.

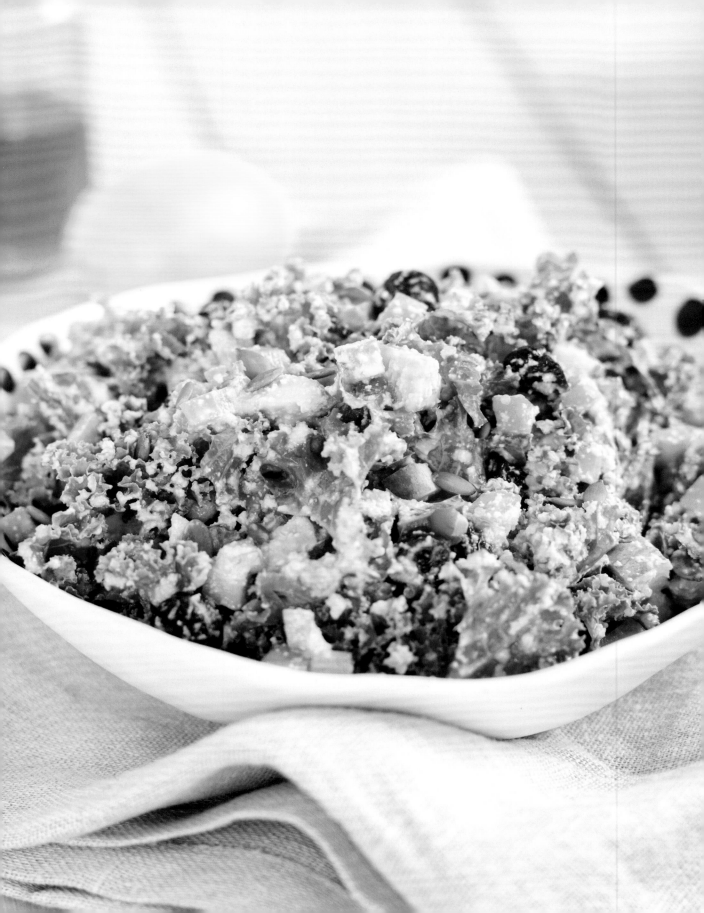

Superfood Salad with Creamy Dressing

I make sure to include this recipe in all my corporate cooking classes because it's easy to make and loved by all. Everyone is shocked that cashews are the secret creamy ingredient in the dressing. I make it at home quite often too because leftovers keep really well for lunch the next day.

Makes 4 servings

 Vegetarian   **Gluten-free**   **Dairy-free**   **Refined Sugar-free**

Creamy Dressing

⅔ cup (150 mL) raw cashews

¾ cup (175 mL) filtered water

¼ cup (60 mL) lemon juice

1½ tsp (7 mL) Dijon mustard

1 tsp (5 mL) liquid honey

1 garlic clove, peeled

Sea salt and pepper to taste

Salad

1 bunch kale, centre stems removed, torn into small bite-size pieces

2 tbsp (30 mL) extra-virgin olive oil

1 cup (250 mL) cooked white quinoa

1 cup (250 mL) finely chopped carrots

2 Gala apples, cored and finely chopped

⅓ cup (75 mL) dried cherries

¼ cup (60 mL) raw pumpkin seeds

Sea salt and pepper

1 avocado, peeled, pitted and cubed

To make the dressing, soak cashews in room-temperature water to cover for at least an hour. Drain.

In a food processor or blender, combine cashews, the ¾ cup (175 mL) water, lemon juice, mustard, honey, garlic, salt and pepper. Blend until smooth.

To make the salad, place torn kale in a large bowl and drizzle with olive oil. Massage with your hands to break down the tough fibre. Add quinoa, carrots, apples, dried cherries and pumpkin seeds. Toss well. Season with sea salt and pepper.

Pour dressing over salad and top with avocado cubes.

> ### *Joyous Tip*
> • • •
> Be careful of some brands of Dijon because they can contain preservatives and additives, just like any condiment. I always buy Dijon from farmers' markets. There is a great Canadian brand I love called Kozlik's.

Cucumber Watermelon Salad

This salad goes perfectly with the Fish "Tacos" with Mango Avocado Salsa on page 223. It's really the perfect summer dinner.

Makes 4 servings

 Vegan   Gluten-free   Dairy-free   Sugar-free

2 cups (500 mL) cubed watermelon

2 cups (500 mL) cubed cucumber

1/2 cup (125 mL) chopped fresh mint

Juice of 2 limes

Sea salt to taste

Toss all ingredients together in a large salad bowl. Serve immediately.

> *Joyous Tip*
>
> • • •
>
> Watermelon and cucumber are two of the most hydrating foods, being over 90 percent water. Eating hydrating foods is as important as drinking plenty of water for weight loss and detoxification to occur.

Avocado Tomato Salsa

When I feel like a quick weekend snack, I often whip this up to enjoy with gluten-free crackers.

Makes 2 servings

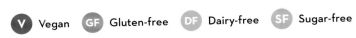 **V** Vegan   **GF** Gluten-free   **DF** Dairy-free   **SF** Sugar-free

1 avocado, peeled, pitted and cut into small chunks

¼ red onion, finely chopped

1 tomato, finely chopped

Juice of 1 lime

Sea salt to taste

Toss all ingredients together in a bowl and enjoy right away.

> ## Joyous Tip
> • • •
> When shopping for a perfectly ripe avocado, simply remove the "button" at the stem end of the avocado to check the colour of the flesh. It should be bright green.

Purple and Green Cabbage Slaw

Cabbage is a crunchy detox superfood and goes perfectly with the Juicy Chicken Spinach Burgers on page 224. You'll love how easy this is to make.

Makes 4 to 6 servings

 Vegetarian   **Gluten-free**   **Dairy-free**   **Refined Sugar-free**

Slaw

½ purple cabbage, cored

½ green cabbage, cored

½ cup (125 mL) shelled hemp seeds

½ cup (125 mL) currants

¼ cup (60 mL) raw pumpkin seeds

¼ cup (60 mL) finely chopped red onion

¼ cup (60 mL) finely chopped fresh cilantro or basil

Dressing

¾ cup (175 mL) extra-virgin olive oil

¼ cup (60 mL) apple cider vinegar

2 tbsp (30 mL) liquid honey

2 tbsp (30 mL) filtered water

To make the salad, shred the cabbage using either a box grater or a food processor. In a large bowl, combine all the salad ingredients.

To make the dressing, combine all ingredients in a bowl (or jar) and whisk (or shake) until emulsified.

Pour dressing over salad, toss, and either let the flavours mingle for an hour or two or enjoy immediately.

> ## Joyous Tip
> • • •
> If you don't have any apple cider vinegar on hand, swap in white wine vinegar or balsamic vinegar.

Crunch-tastic Sauerkraut

This recipe comes from the fermentation goddess Kathrin, a fellow holistic nutritionist and owner of For Love of Body. She has been teaching workshops on fermentation for years. This crunchy sauerkraut is a rich source of prebiotics and easy-to-absorb nutrients.

Fills 1 wide-mouth quart (1 L) mason jar or 2 wide-mouth pint (500 mL) mason jars

 Vegan   **Gluten-free**   **Dairy-free**   **Sugar-free**

1 large purple or green cabbage

1 to 2 tbsp (15 to 30 mL) sea salt

4 carrots

1 tart apple, such as Granny Smith

Set aside a few outer leaves of the cabbage. Shred or chop the rest of the cabbage (you can use the shredder disc on a food processor to speed things up) and place in a large bowl. Sprinkle with sea salt (use the larger amount for a crunchier sauerkraut). Roll up your sleeves and massage kraut with your hands for a few minutes, until cabbage begins to soften and release water.

Coarsely grate or julienne carrots and apple and add to cabbage. Mix well.

Begin to stuff mixture into clean glass jars. Push down with your clean hands or a wooden spoon or mallet, getting rid of any air bubbles and helping to push more water out of the cabbage. Keep pushing and packing until the released water covers the kraut. (You may need to let it sit for a little while to let the cabbage release enough water.)

Pack jars as tightly as possible to within 2 inches (5 cm) of the rim. Once enough water has released to cover the veggies, use your reserved cabbage leaves to push the veggies down into the water. (This is important! Keeping the veggies submerged lets good bacteria ferment and keeps bad bacteria out.)

Top with a lid, but don't tighten completely, as you need to let air from the fermentation process escape. Set in warm place, out of direct light, for 2 to 7 days, depending on how warm the kitchen is (the warmer the room, the less time fermentation will take). Begin tasting after 2 days. Once it's tangy to your liking, discard the top cabbage leaf, close lid tightly and transfer to the fridge, where it will keep for several months.

> ## Joyous Tip
>
> • • •
>
> In the first few days, you will see air bubbles rising. This is a good sign! But if the bubbling causes liquid to spill over, set jars on a shallow plate.
>
> If the cabbage doesn't exude enough water to submerge everything, you will need to add some brine (salted water). Dissolve 1½ tsp (7 mL) of sea salt per cup (250 mL) of water and add enough brine to cover the kraut.
>
> If you see foam forming on top, this is normal. Just spoon it off.

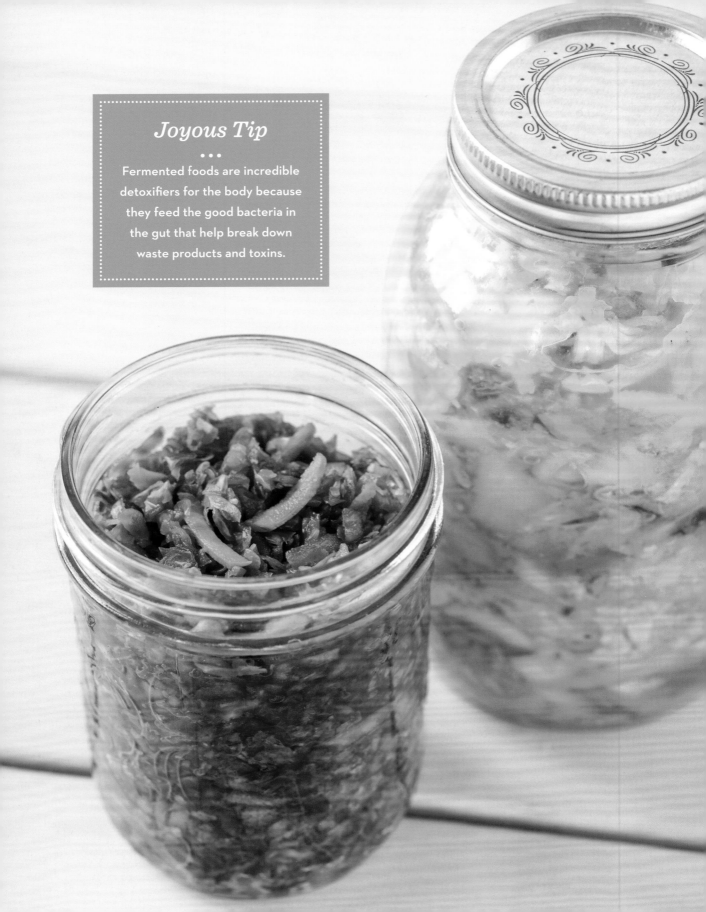

Spring-Inspired Kimchi

This recipe was created by the fermentation goddess Kathrin (see page 205). My favourite way to eat kimchi is with eggs, though it works well as a condiment for just about anything. Enjoy this kimchi with the Family Veggie Frittata on page 109.

Fills 1 wide-mouth quart (1 L) mason jar or 2 wide-mouth pint (500 mL) mason jars

 Vegan Gluten-free Dairy-free Sugar-free

1 napa cabbage, cored and coarsely chopped,
    1 large leaf reserved

3 carrots, grated

3 or 4 red radishes, thinly sliced

1 bunch green onions, chopped

2 tbsp (30 mL) sea salt

Paste

2 to 4 garlic cloves, peeled

1-inch (2.5 cm) piece fresh ginger, grated

1 pear, cored and chopped

2 to 4 tbsp (30 to 60 mL) red chili flakes
    (depending on how hot you like it)

If your carrots and pear are not organic, then peel them. Combine cabbage, carrots, radishes and green onions in a large bowl. Set aside.

To make the paste, place garlic, ginger, pear and chili flakes in a food processor or blender. Pulse until combined and fairly smooth.

Pour paste over vegetable mixture, then sprinkle with sea salt. Using your hands, massage kimchi. (You can use gloves for this if you prefer; there's heat from the ginger and chili flakes.) As you massage, the veggies will start to soften and release water, creating a brine. You can take breaks if you like, allowing kimchi to sit and release brine, then come back and massage a bit more. You need to create enough brine to cover the kimchi when you stuff it into the jar, so there should be a good puddle at the bottom of the bowl.

Once you have enough brine, begin to stuff kimchi and brine into a clean mason jar. Use a wooden spoon or mallet to push down on kimchi to remove air pockets and release more water. Leave 1 to 2 inches (2.5 to 5 cm) of space from the rim of the jar, then top with the reserved cabbage leaf, using it to push down the kimchi so it is submerged under the brine.

Screw the lid on loosely so that air can still escape and leave to ferment. This will take 7 to 10 days, depending on the temperature of the kitchen. Check your kimchi daily. If necessary, push the leaf on top down to keep vegetables submerged under the brine. Begin tasting after a week. Once fermented to your liking (it will be slightly tangy and the cabbage will be soft), remove the top cabbage leaf, close lid tightly and store in the fridge, where it will keep for several months.

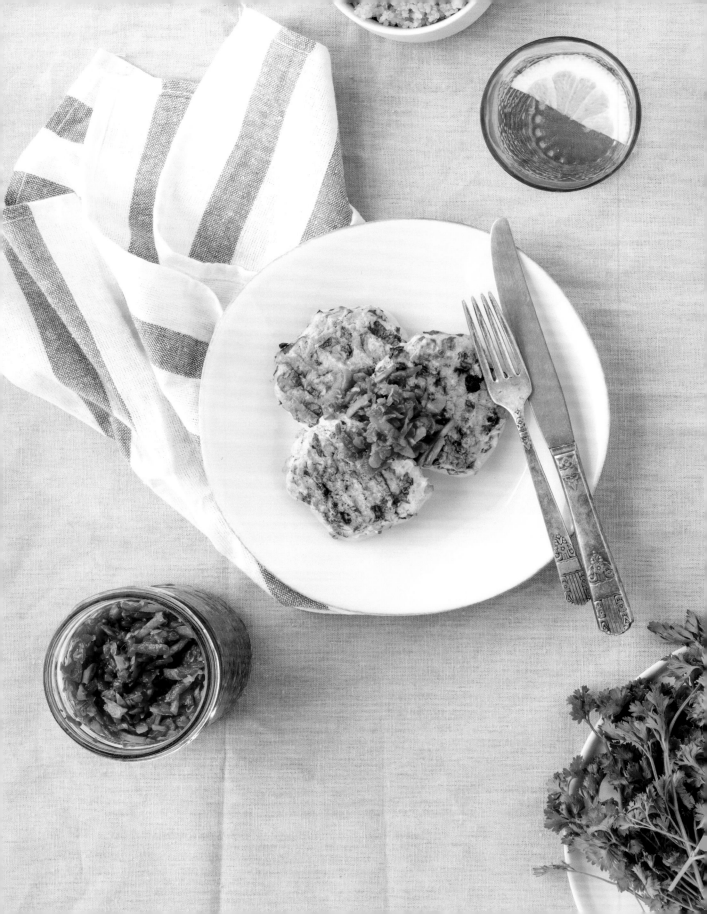

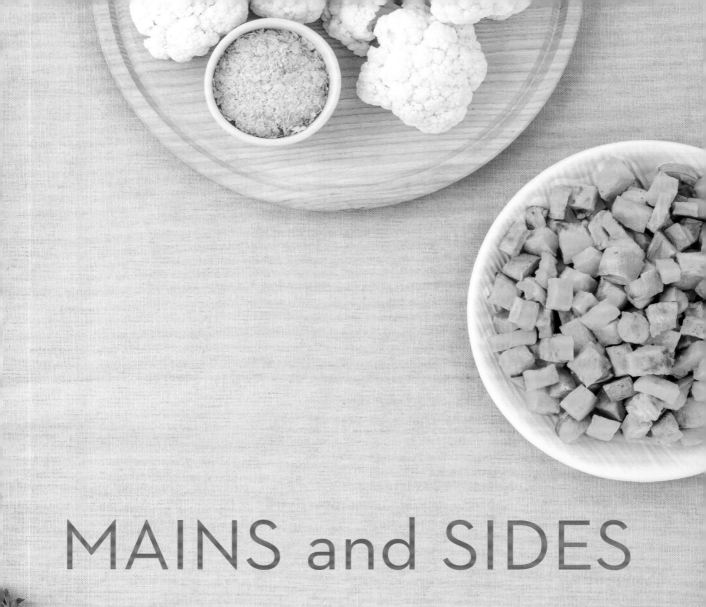

MAINS and SIDES

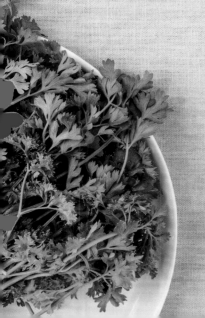

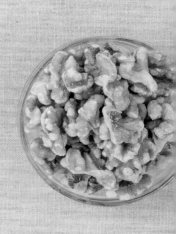

Baked Mac and Cheese

My husband, Walker, and I enjoy this one-pot dish because it lasts over a couple of nights. It's super convenient when we have a busy week because it reheats easily. And it's so full of flavour, you won't even miss the dairy-filled version. This dish goes really well with the Chopped Kale and Beet Salad on page 183.

Makes 4 servings

 Vegan   Gluten-free   Dairy-free   Sugar-free

1 cup (250 mL) raw cashews

1/2 cup (125 mL) grated carrot

1 cup (250 mL) boiling water

1/4 cup (60 mL) nutritional yeast

2 tbsp (30 mL) Dijon mustard (grainy or smooth)

1 tsp (5 mL) apple cider vinegar

1 garlic clove, minced

Sea salt and pepper to taste

2 cups (500 mL) gluten-free macaroni (brown rice or quinoa pasta)

1/2 medium red onion, finely chopped

1 or 2 medium tomatoes, chopped

1/4 cup (60 mL) shelled hemp seeds

Soak cashews in enough water to cover for 4 hours. Drain.

Preheat oven to 350°F (180°C).

To make the cheese sauce, in a blender or food processor, combine cashews, carrot and boiling water. Blend until smooth. Add nutritional yeast, mustard, cider vinegar, garlic, sea salt and pepper. Purée until creamy. Set aside.

Bring a large pot of water to a boil. Add macaroni and cook until tender but still chewy. Drain. Return hot pasta to the pot, add red onion, tomatoes and cheese sauce and combine well. Spread mixture evenly in an 8-inch (2 L) square baking dish. Bake for 15 minutes or until top is golden brown. Sprinkle with hemp seeds and serve hot.

Joyous Tip

• • •

Nutritional yeast is deactivated yeast. It's sold either flaked or as a powder and it has a parmesan-like flavour. It contains trace amounts of nutrients and is often fortified with vitamin B_{12}. I would suggest purchasing certified organic. You can find it in health food stores and many grocery stores. If you want a cheesier mac and cheese, use less macaroni.

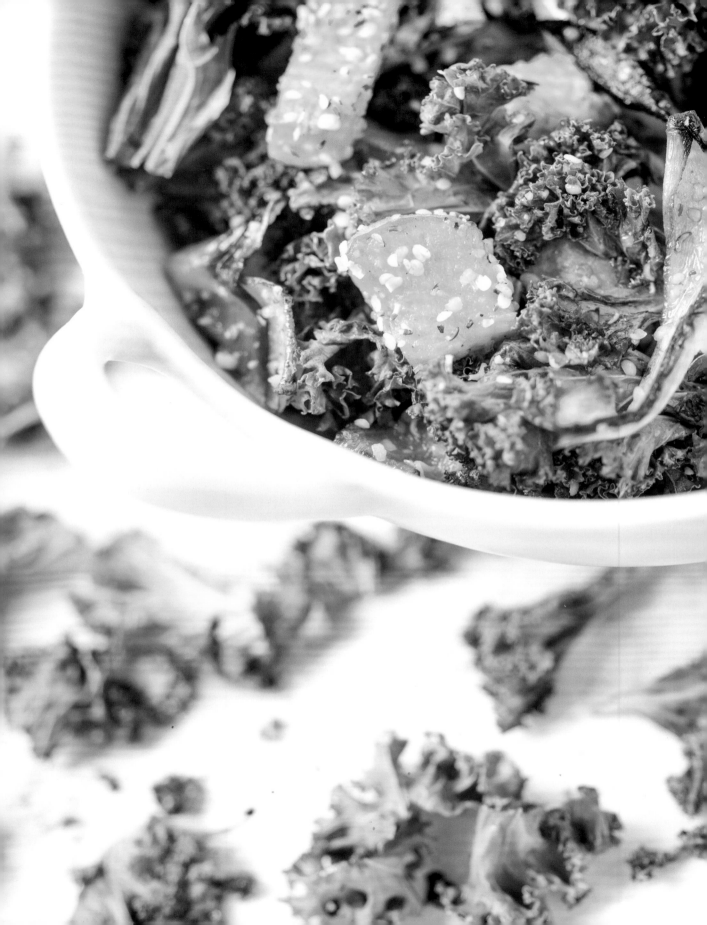

Warm Sweet Potato Kale Bowl with Quinoa

This recipe has been a *Joyous Health* blog reader favourite for years. Kale is a detox superfood, and sweet potatoes are the perfect comfort food, so combining them together in this wonderful dish just made sense! I hope it becomes a favourite of yours too.

Makes 2 to 4 servings

 Vegan   Gluten-free   Dairy-free   Sugar-free

2 sweet potatoes (unpeeled if organic), chopped into small cubes

½ red onion, finely chopped

2 tbsp (30 mL) extra-virgin olive oil, plus more for drizzling

Sea salt and pepper

6 large kale leaves, centre stems removed, cut into bite-size pieces

1 tbsp (15 mL) balsamic vinegar

1 cup (250 mL) cooked white quinoa

1 tbsp (15 mL) sesame seeds

Preheat oven to 375°F (190°C).

In a bowl, toss sweet potatoes and onion in 1 tbsp (15 mL) of the olive oil. Spread evenly on a parchment-lined baking sheet and season with sea salt and pepper. (Set aside the bowl.) Bake for 25 to 30 minutes, until the potatoes are fork-tender. Return sweet potatoes and onions to the bowl.

Reduce oven temperature to 350°F (180°C). Spread kale on the same baking sheet and drizzle with balsamic vinegar and the remaining 1 tbsp (15 mL) olive oil. Bake for 6 to 8 minutes, until kale is slightly crispy on the edges. Watch closely because it burns easily. (You can cook the kale at the same time as the sweet potatoes if you like, but it will cook in less time because of the higher temperature.)

Add kale and quinoa to the sweet potatoes and mix together. Drizzle with extra-virgin olive oil, season with sea salt and pepper and sprinkle with sesame seeds.

> ## *Joyous Tip*
> • • •
> If you don't have any quinoa on hand, use shelled hemp seeds instead. They are super convenient because they don't require cooking! You can watch a step-by-step video of this recipe on my YouTube channel, joyoushealth1.

Cheesy Cauliflower Casserole

If you loved the Baked Mac and Cheese on page 211 but prefer something grain-free, then you'll love this pasta-free makeover.

Serves 4 to 6 as a side dish

 Vegan   **Gluten-free**   **Dairy-free**   **Sugar-free**

1 cup (250 mL) raw cashews

½ cup (125 mL) grated carrot

1 cup (250 mL) boiling water

1 white onion, finely chopped

3 garlic cloves, minced

⅓ cup (75 mL) nutritional yeast

2 tbsp (30 mL) Dijon mustard

1 tsp (5 mL) apple cider vinegar

½ tsp (2 mL) cayenne pepper

Sea salt and black pepper to taste

1 head cauliflower, chopped into bite-size pieces

Soak cashews in enough water to cover for 4 hours. Drain.

Preheat oven to 350°F (180°C).

To make the cheese sauce, in a blender or food processor, combine cashews, carrot and boiling water. Blend until smooth. Add onions, garlic, nutritional yeast, mustard, cider vinegar, cayenne, sea salt and pepper. Purée until creamy. Set aside.

Bring a large pot of water to a boil. Add cauliflower and boil for 6 to 7 minutes, until it is fork-tender but not mushy. Drain. (You can also steam the cauliflower if you prefer.)

In a large bowl, stir together cauliflower and cheese sauce. Spoon into a 10-inch (3 L) square baking dish. Bake for 15 minutes. Serve hot.

> *Joyous Tip*
>
> • • •
>
> Cauliflower is a detox superfood. It shares with broccoli, kale and cabbage a variety of phytonutrients that support detoxification of the liver. These foods are often referred to as "anti-cancer powerfoods."

Cauliflower Rice

If you ever get bored of brown rice as a side dish, or you find grains bothersome to your digestion, then you'll love this delicious, super-easy alternative. It goes well with pretty much any dish. Cauliflower is a detox superfood.

Makes 4 servings

 Vegan **Gluten-free** **Dairy-free** **SF** **Sugar-free**

1 head cauliflower, cut into large chunks

2 tbsp (30 mL) extra-virgin olive oil

1 large white onion, finely chopped

2 garlic cloves, chopped

1/2 cup (125 mL) vegetable stock or filtered water

1 tsp (5 mL) sea salt

1/2 tsp (2 mL) freshly ground black pepper

Nutritional yeast (optional)

Chopped fresh herbs (optional)

Using the grating disc of your food processor (or a box grater), grate cauliflower into fine bits. It should be similar to white rice in size.

Heat olive oil in a large saucepan over medium heat. Add onions and garlic and cook, stirring frequently, for 4 to 6 minutes. Add the cauliflower and cook for another 6 minutes.

Add stock and continue to cook until cauliflower is tender, approximately 15 minutes. Season with sea salt and pepper. If using, add nutritional yeast and fresh herbs.

Chickpea Burgers

This is a *Joyous Health* blog reader favourite and my "go-to" veggie burger when I want a fast, healthy meal. They taste just as good chilled, so I often pack them for lunch the next day along with a big green salad. They are delicious served with the Superfood Salad with Creamy Dressing on page 201.

Makes 8 small patties

 Vegetarian   **Gluten-free**   **Dairy-free**   **SF** **Sugar-free**

1 can (15 oz/425 g) chickpeas, drained and rinsed

½ cup (125 mL) almond meal/flour (ground almonds)

½ cup (125 mL) ground chia, ground flax seeds or a mixture

½ cup (125 mL) grated carrots

¼ cup (60 mL) diced red onion

¼ cup (60 mL) chopped fresh parsley

¼ cup (60 mL) chopped fresh basil

2 tbsp (30 mL) extra-virgin olive oil

1 tsp (5 mL) cayenne pepper or red chili flakes

2 eggs (or egg substitution, page 81)

Pinch of sea salt and pepper

Sliced green onions, for garnish

Toss all ingredients except green onions into a food processor and blend into a paste. The mixture will be sticky. Shape mixture into 8 patties.

You have three options for cooking:

1.   Heat a grill to medium and cook for 5 to 7 minutes on each side (see tip).

2.   Melt 1 tbsp (15 mL) coconut oil in a large skillet. Cook for 5 to 7 minutes on each side or until golden brown.

3.   Roll mixture into balls and bake them at 350°F (180°C) for 15 to 20 minutes, like baked falafel.

Top burgers with sliced green onions and a drizzle of extra-virgin olive oil. Serve with a beautiful raw leafy green salad and some sliced ripe avocado.

> ## *Joyous Tip*
> • • •
> Buy BPA-free canned beans if you are not cooking them yourself.
> These burgers cook best on an indoor grill, because the
> lid helps them stick together really well.

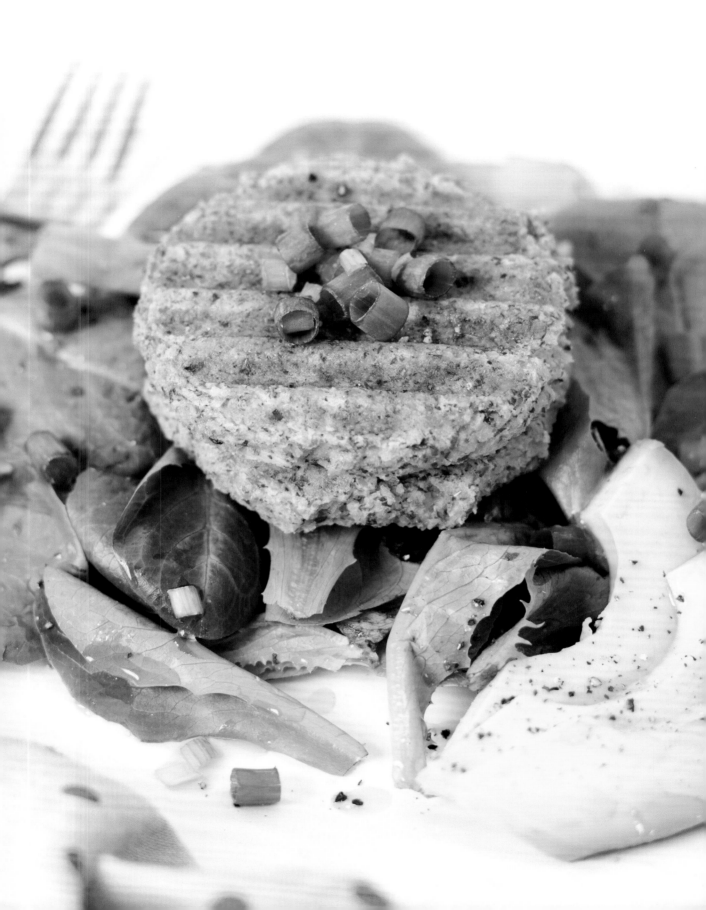

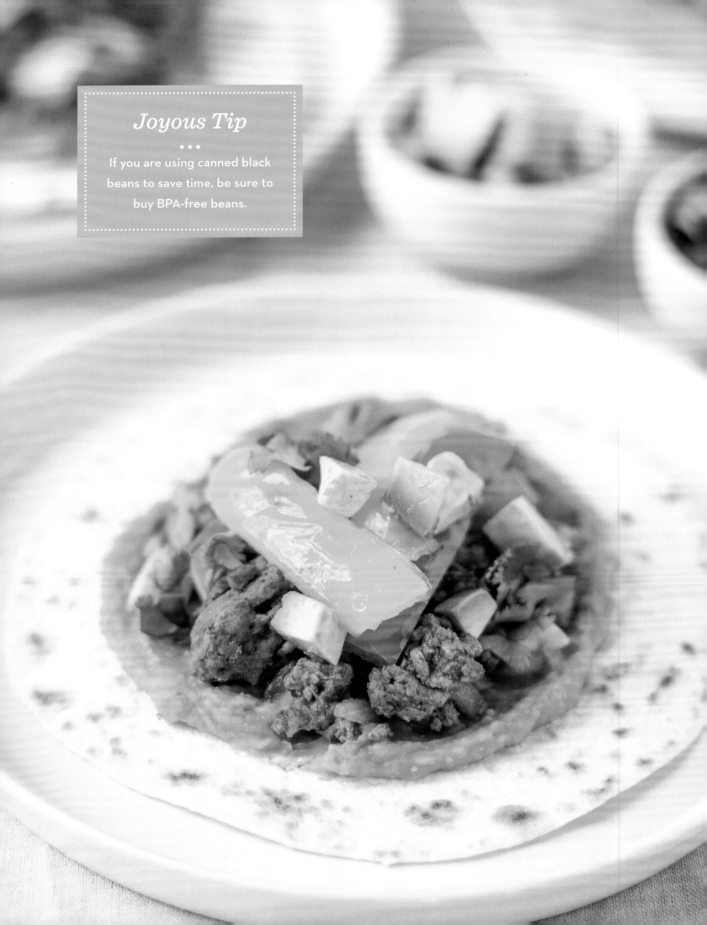

Joyous Tip

• • •

If you are using canned black
beans to save time, be sure to
buy BPA-free beans.

Spicy Cacao Chicken Tortillas

Cacao and chicken might seem an odd pairing, but the chocolate flavour is not overpowering. It's the perfect combo of sweet and savoury, and it's become a favourite in my family.

Makes 4 servings

 Gluten-free   Dairy-free   Sugar-free

2 sweet peppers (any colour), thinly sliced

1 zucchini, thinly sliced

2 tbsp (30 mL) extra-virgin olive oil

Sea salt and black pepper

½ lb (225 g) ground chicken or turkey (preferably organic)

1 medium red onion, finely chopped

3 garlic cloves, minced

3 tbsp (45 mL) raw cacao powder or unsweetened cocoa powder

1 tsp (5 mL) ground cumin

1 tsp (5 mL) chili powder

½ to 1 tsp (2 to 5 mL) cayenne pepper (depending how spicy you like it)

1 tsp (5 mL) dried Italian herbs

1 cup (250 mL) cooked black beans

2 tbsp (30 mL) filtered water

8 small brown rice tortillas

1 avocado, peeled, pitted and diced

⅓ cup (75 mL) chopped fresh cilantro

1 lime

Preheat oven to 375°F (190°C).

Toss bell peppers and zucchini with 1 tbsp (15 mL) of the olive oil and sea salt and black pepper to taste. Spread on a parchment-lined baking sheet. Roast for 15 to 20 minutes or until vegetables are tender. You don't need to stir them. Set aside.

Heat remaining 1 tbsp (15 mL) oil in a large saucepan over medium heat. Add chicken, onions, garlic, cacao, cumin, chili powder, cayenne, dried herbs and sea salt to taste. Cook, stirring frequently, until no pink is visible in the chicken, approximately 15 minutes. Remove from heat.

Meanwhile, in a small saucepan, combine black beans and water. Warm them over low heat, mashing them with a fork or toss into a food processor and blend until a paste.

To assemble, spread beans on tortillas and top with chicken mixture, vegetable mixture, avocado and cilantro. Squirt with some lime juice.

Option: You can heat the tortillas to make them crispy. Heat about ½ tsp (2 mL) olive oil in a skillet over medium heat. Cook tortillas for about 3 minutes on each side, until golden brown.

Mint Guacamole Lettuce Wraps

I love easy-peasy meals that don't require me to turn on an oven or use the stovetop, especially in the heat of summer. These wraps can be a side dish or the main event—perfect for cottage weekends! You can bump up the protein by adding more hemp seeds if you like.

Makes 6 to 8 lettuce wraps

 Vegan   Gluten-free   Dairy-free   Sugar-free

4 avocados, peeled and pitted

Juice of 3 limes

¼ cup (60 mL) packed chopped fresh mint

½ sweet red pepper, finely chopped

1 tomato, finely chopped

½ red onion, finely chopped

⅓ to ½ cup (75 to 125 mL) shelled hemp seeds

1 to 2 garlic cloves, minced

½ tsp (2 mL) sea salt

8 romaine lettuce leaves

In a large bowl, mash together avocados and lime juice with a fork. Add mint, red pepper, tomato, onion, hemp seeds, garlic and sea salt. Spoon mint guacamole into lettuce leaves.

> *Joyous Tip*
>
> • • •
>
> You can find shelled hemp seeds (hemp hearts) in the natural foods section of the grocery store or at health food stores.

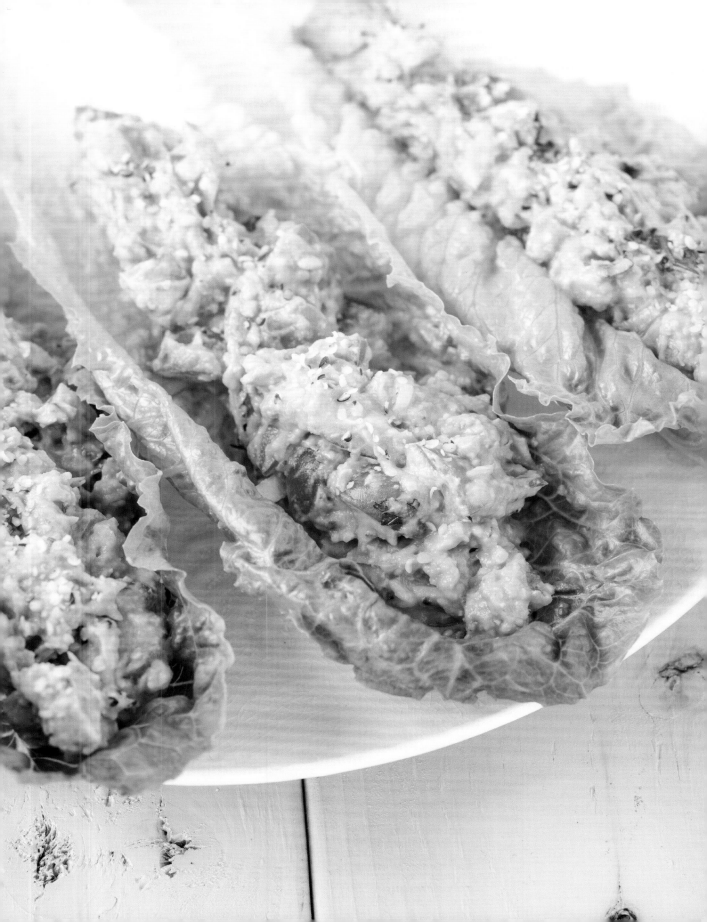

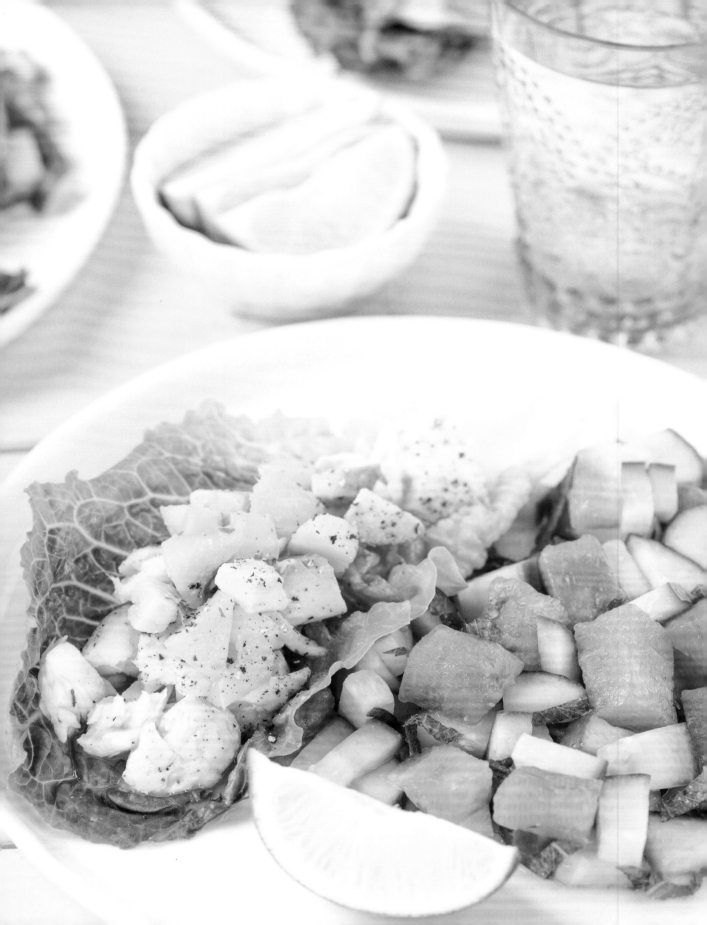

Fish "Tacos" with Mango Avocado Salsa

Walker and I love all things Mexican, including tacos. This dish is a fresh, vibrant meal full of detox-friendly foods. These lettuce "tacos" are delicious served with the Cucumber Watermelon Salad on page 202. It's also a great dish if you are entertaining because it's so easy to make and everyone always loves it.

Makes 4 servings

 Gluten-free   **Dairy-free**   **Sugar-free**

4 white flaky fish fillets (such as cod, tilapia or sole)

⅓ cup (75 mL) lime juice

¼ cup (60 mL) extra-virgin olive oil

Sea salt and pepper

¼ tsp (1 mL) cayenne pepper (optional)

8 romaine lettuce leaves

Mango Avocado Salsa

2 avocados, peeled, pitted and cubed

2 ripe mangoes, peeled and cubed

½ cup (125 mL) chopped fresh cilantro

Juice of 2 limes (reserve some to squirt over assembled tacos)

Pinch of sea salt

Preheat oven to 350°F (180°C).

In a shallow baking dish, arrange fish skin side down. Stir together lime juice and olive oil. Pour over fish. Season with sea salt, pepper and cayenne, if using. Bake for 20 to 25 minutes, until fish is fully cooked and flaky.

Meanwhile, in a medium bowl, combine all the salsa ingredients. Set aside to let the flavours mingle.

To assemble, place flaked fish on romaine leaves and top with salsa. Finish with a squirt of lime juice.

> ## *Joyous Tip*
> • • •
> Avoid farm-raised tilapia from China. A 2009 study conducted for the U.S. Department of Agriculture cited some alarming facts about Chinese farm-raised seafood. Researchers noted that "many of China's farms and food processors are situated in heavily industrialized regions where water, air and soil are contaminated by industrial effluents and vehicle exhaust."

Juicy Chicken Spinach Burgers

Burgers aren't just for summer BBQs. I make them all year round, as they are the perfect protein accompaniment to any side dish or salad. I highly recommend these with the Purple and Green Cabbage Slaw on page 204.

Makes 4 to 6 servings

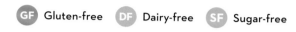 **GF** Gluten-free   **DF** Dairy-free   **SF** Sugar-free

1 lb (450 g) ground organic chicken

¹/₂ onion, finely chopped

³/₄ cup (175 mL) chopped fresh spinach

¹/₂ cup (125 mL) loosely packed chopped fresh cilantro

1 tbsp (15 mL) gluten-free tamari sauce

1 tsp (5 mL) cayenne pepper

1 tsp (5 mL) garlic powder (or 2 garlic cloves, minced)

¹/₂ tsp (2 mL) sea salt

Combine all ingredients in a large bowl. Mix gently but thoroughly. Let sit for 30 minutes in the fridge for the flavours to mingle.

Heat an indoor grill to medium. Shape chicken mixture into 4 to 6 burgers. Grill burgers for 10 to 12 minutes or until there is no pink in the middle. If your grill has a lid, you may need to reduce the cooking time.

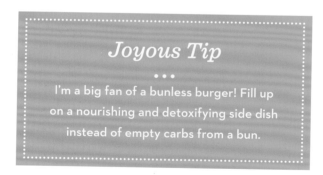

Joyous Tip

• • •

I'm a big fan of a bunless burger! Fill up on a nourishing and detoxifying side dish instead of empty carbs from a bun.

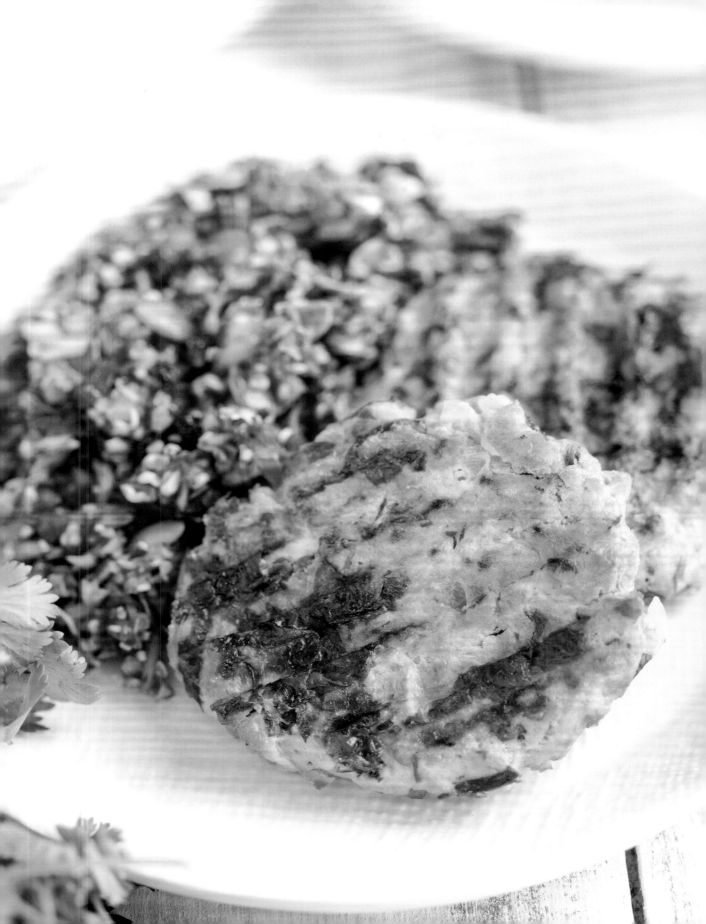

Roasted Balsamic Kale

If you're not a fan of raw kale, then you'll love this roasted version of my all-time favourite detox superfood. The balsamic vinegar softens the bitterness of the kale. It is so versatile it can accompany any protein, from fish to chicken to grilled tempeh.

Makes 2 servings

 Vegan   Gluten-free   Dairy-free   Sugar-free

1 bunch lacinato or curly kale, centre stems removed

1 tbsp (15 mL) balsamic vinegar

1½ tsp (7 mL) extra-virgin olive oil

Pinch of sea salt

Preheat oven to 350°F (180°C).

Tear kale into bite-size pieces. Place on a baking sheet, drizzle with vinegar and olive oil and sprinkle with sea salt. Massage the kale with your hands to make sure the oil and vinegar are well distributed. Spread kale into an even layer.

Bake for 8 minutes or until kale is soft but not crispy. Watch closely as it can burn easily.

Grilled Tempeh Kebabs with the Best Ever Homemade BBQ Sauce

The BBQ sauce adds a ton of flavour to these tempeh kebabs. They are the perfect dish for summer entertaining, and none of your guests will miss the hamburgers or steak! Enjoy them with chopped crunchy vegetables and Creamy Cashew Veggie Dip on page 193.

Makes 4 servings

 Vegan   Gluten-free   Dairy-free   Refined Sugar-free

Best Ever Homemade BBQ Sauce

1 can (5.5 oz/156 mL) tomato paste

1/4 cup (60 mL) real maple syrup

1/4 cup (60 mL) gluten-free tamari sauce

3 tbsp (45 mL) Dijon mustard

3 tbsp (45 mL) apple cider vinegar

1 1/2 tsp (7 mL) garlic powder

1 1/2 tsp (7 mL) onion powder

1/2 tsp (2 mL) sea salt

Freshly ground pepper

Kebabs

1 lb (450 g) tempeh, cut into 1 1/2-inch (4 cm) cubes

1 sweet red or yellow pepper, cut into bite-size chunks

1 red onion, cut into bite-size chunks

1 zucchini, sliced 1 inch (2.5 cm) thick

To make the BBQ sauce, combine all ingredients in a medium bowl and stir together well.

To make the kebabs, in a large bowl, combine all ingredients. Coat with BBQ sauce, reserving some sauce for serving. Marinate for a few hours or overnight.

Divide tempeh and vegetables evenly onto skewers, alternating ingredients.

Heat a grill to medium. Grill kebabs, turning occasionally, for 7 to 10 minutes or until the vegetables are tender. (You can also bake these kebabs in a baking dish for 25 minutes at 350°F/180°C.) Serve immediately with remaining BBQ sauce.

> ## *Joyous Tip*
> • • •
> Tempeh is made from fermented soybeans. It is rich in protein and fibre.
> It has a mild flavour and takes on the flavours of what you cook it with.
> Be sure to purchase certified organic tempeh to avoid GMO soybeans.

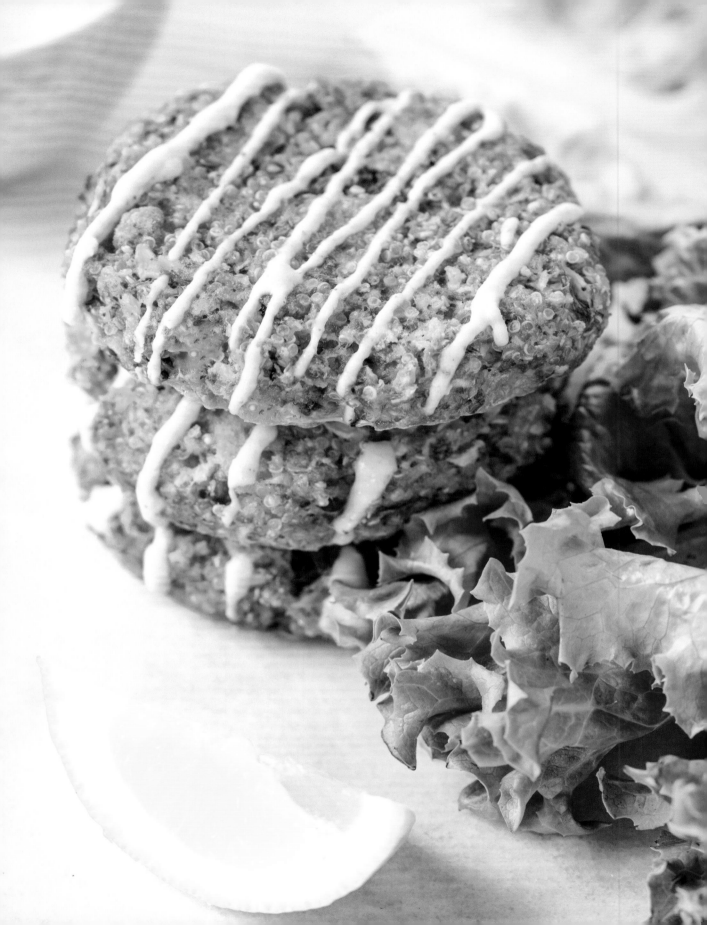

Salmon Quinoa Cakes with Lemon Sauce

The first time I ever made these salmon cakes and posted them on Instagram, everyone was clamouring for the recipe because they are as pretty as they are delicious! These go really nicely with the Refreshing Sweet Pea Soup on page 166.

Makes 4 or 5 cakes

 Gluten-free   **Dairy-free**   **SF** **Sugar-free**

Lemon Tahini Sauce

2 tbsp (30 mL) tahini

1 tbsp (15 mL) Dijon mustard

Juice of 1 lemon

1 tbsp (15 mL) filtered water

Quinoa Cakes

1/2 cup (125 mL) white quinoa

1 cup (250 mL) filtered water

1 can (7.5 oz/213 g) wild salmon
   (or 1 cooked fish fillet, flaked)

1 carrot, grated

2 green onions, finely chopped

2 eggs

1/4 cup (60 mL) chopped fresh herbs
   (choose your favourite)

2 tbsp (30 mL) Dijon mustard

2 tbsp (30 mL) ground flaxseeds

1/2 tsp (2 mL) garlic powder (or 1 clove garlic, minced)

Pinch of sea salt and pepper

Preheat oven to 350°F (180°C).

To make the lemon tahini sauce, place all ingredients in a food processor or blender and blend until creamy. If sauce is too thick, add a little more water. Set aside.

To cook the quinoa, combine water and quinoa in a medium pot and bring to a boil. Cover, reduce heat to low and simmer for 15 minutes or until quinoa is fluffy.

In a medium bowl, combine quinoa, salmon, carrot, green onions, eggs, fresh herbs, mustard, flaxseeds, garlic powder, sea salt and pepper. Mix well. Shape into 4 or 5 patties about 3/4 inch (2 cm) thick. Arrange on a parchment-lined baking sheet. Cook for 22 minutes or until golden. Serve drizzled with the lemon tahini sauce.

> ## *Joyous Tip*
> • • •
> Some brands of quinoa require you to rinse before cooking and then rinse again after cooking to remove any bitter saponins. If your quinoa is labelled "pre-washed," you can skip this step. For a step-by-step video of this recipe, visit joyoushealth.com/quinoacakes.

Sesame Orange Quinoa Bowl

The first time I ever made this was for a girlfriend's bachelorette party, and it was a huge hit. I knew this by the number of emails I received in the next few days asking me for the recipe. The dressing is the hero of this dish, so you might want to double it and have it on hand for other uses.

Serves 4 to 6 as a side dish

 Vegetarian   Gluten-free   Dairy-free   Refined Sugar-free

1½ cups (375 mL) white quinoa

3 cups (750 mL) filtered water

3 or 4 roasted sweet potatoes, cut into small chunks.

2 cups (500 mL) loosely packed fresh spinach

3 green onions, chopped

2 handfuls of chopped fresh parsley, cilantro or other green herb

2 tbsp (30 mL) sesame seeds, for garnish

Dressing

¼ cup (60 mL) white wine vinegar

2 tbsp (30 mL) sesame oil

¼ cup (60 mL) liquid honey

¼ cup (60 mL) gluten-free tamari sauce

1 tbsp (15 mL) minced peeled fresh ginger

Zest of 1 orange (if organic)

Juice of 2 large oranges

Combine quinoa and water in a medium pot and bring to a boil. Cover, reduce heat to low and simmer for 15 minutes or until quinoa is fluffy.

Meanwhile, make the dressing. Combine all ingredients in a small bowl; whisk together well. Taste and add more of whatever you feel it needs. Set aside.

In a large bowl, toss together quinoa, sweet potatoes, spinach, green onions and herbs.

Pour over dressing just before serving. Garnish with sesame seeds.

> ## *Joyous Tip*
> • • •
> Leave the skin on the potatoes if they're organic. Much of the fibre and many minerals, including blood sugar balancing chromium, are contained within the skin.

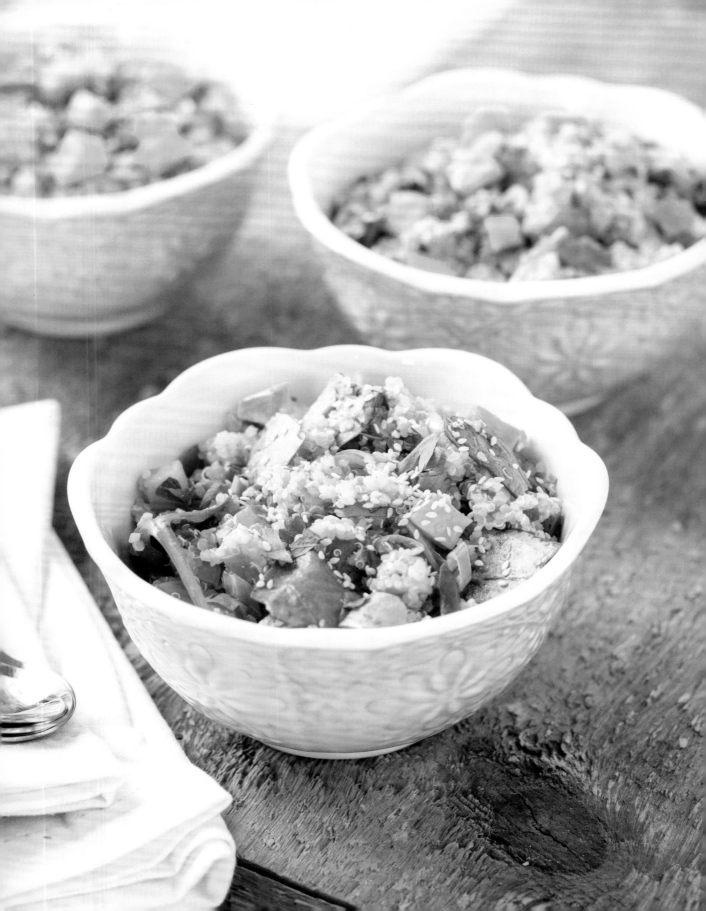

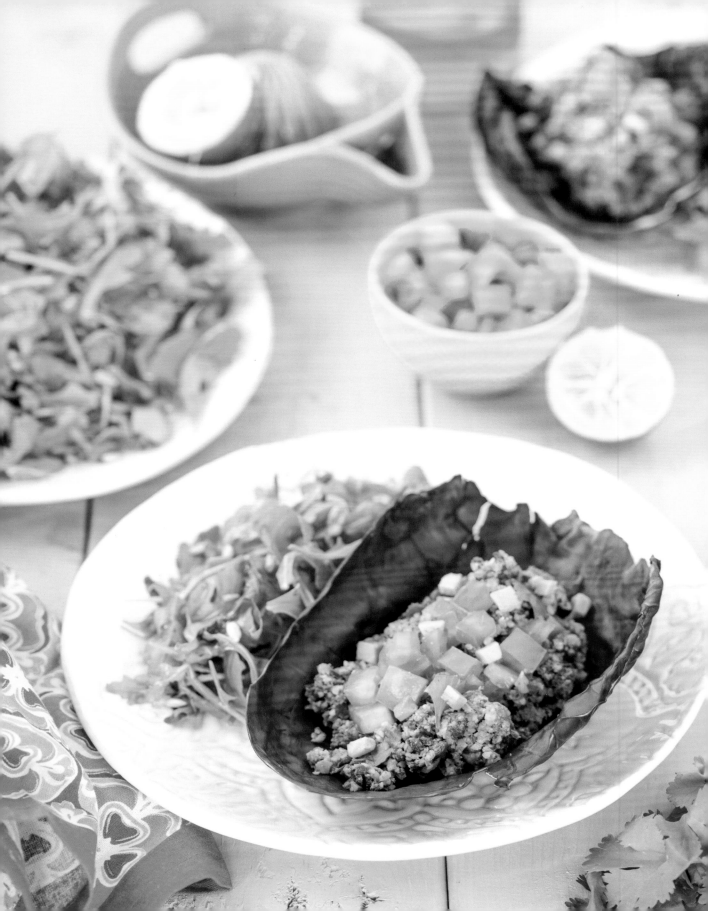

Purple Cabbage Walnut Meat "Tacos"

One of my nutritionist friends, Heather Allen, graciously contributed this recipe to the Joyous 10-Day Detox on my website. I revamped it a bit for this book because it was such a hit. Don't worry, you won't miss animal meat at all, because the walnuts are a wonderful substitute.

Makes 10 to 12 tacos

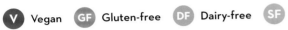 **Vegan** **Gluten-free** **Dairy-free** **Sugar-free**

Walnut Meat

½ cup (125 mL) dry-packed sun-dried tomatoes

1 cup (250 mL) walnuts

1 cup (250 mL) coarsely chopped white button or cremini mushrooms

1 tsp (5 mL) ground cumin

½ tsp (2 mL) garlic powder

¼ tsp (1 mL) chili powder

Pinch of cayenne pepper

Tacos

½ cup (125 mL) chopped tomatoes

¼ cup (60 mL) chopped fresh cilantro

¼ cup (60 mL) diced red onion

2 tbsp (30 mL) lime juice

Pinch of sea salt and pepper

10 to 12 purple cabbage leaves

1 avocado, peeled, pitted and diced

Garnishes: Chopped fresh cilantro, chopped red onion, lime juice, hot sauce

In a small bowl, soak sun-dried tomatoes in hot water to cover for 20 minutes or until soft. Drain and set aside.

Meanwhile, in a medium bowl, combine chopped tomatoes, cilantro, red onion, lime juice, sea salt and pepper. Stir until combined. Set aside.

To make the walnut meat, in a food processor, place sun-dried tomatoes, walnuts, mushrooms, cumin, garlic powder, chili powder and cayenne. Pulse until combined but still chunky. Do not over-process or the mixture will be pasty.

Spoon walnut mixture onto cabbage leaves. Top with tomato mixture and diced avocado. Top with extra cilantro, lime juice, red onions or your favourite hot sauce to kick things up a notch.

Portobello Mushroom Pizza Two Ways

One of my favourite meals, whether I'm detoxing or not, is pizza. Many people assume that pizza is unhealthy, but these two versions are full of flavour and super healthy. Plus, they're full of detox-friendly foods.

Each recipe makes 3 mushroom pizzas

 Vegan   Gluten-free   Dairy-free   Sugar-free

Arugula Pesto Pizza

3 portobello mushrooms, stems removed

Almond Arugula Lemon Pesto (page 196)

½ sweet yellow pepper, thinly sliced

5 or 6 white button or cremini mushrooms, sliced

1 to 2 tbsp (15 to 30 mL) nutritional yeast

Spread pesto on underside of each portobello mushroom. Evenly divide remaining toppings among 3 portobellos.

Preheat oven to 375°F (190°C).

Place portobello pizzas on a parchment-lined baking sheet. Bake for 20 to 25 minutes, until hot. Serve hot, drizzled with extra-virgin olive oil.

Tomato Green Pepper Pizza

3 portobello mushrooms, stems removed

1/2 cup (125 mL) tomato sauce (or 1 tomato, sliced and blended to a paste)

1/2 sweet green pepper, thinly sliced

5 or 6 cherry or grape tomatoes, halved

1/4 red onion, thinly sliced

1/2 hot chili pepper, thinly sliced (or 1 tbsp/15 mL red chili flakes)

1 tsp (5 mL) dried basil

Sea salt and pepper to taste

Spread tomato sauce on underside of each portobello mushroom. Evenly divide remaining toppings among 3 portobellos.

Preheat oven to 375°F (190°C).

Place portobello pizzas on a parchment-lined baking sheet. Bake for 20 to 25 minutes, until hot. Serve hot, drizzled with extra-virgin olive oil.

Joyous Tip

• • •

The mushrooms become very moist when baked, so these pizzas are best eaten with a knife and fork. However, you can reduce their moistness by following these steps:

1. Form a piece of foil into a doughnut shape about 4 inches (10 cm) wide and 1½ inches (4 cm) high. Make 1 ring for each pizza.

2. Place the foil rings on the parchment-lined baking sheet and position the mushroom pizzas on top. Now, all the juices will drain off the mushrooms and they won't sit in their own juices.

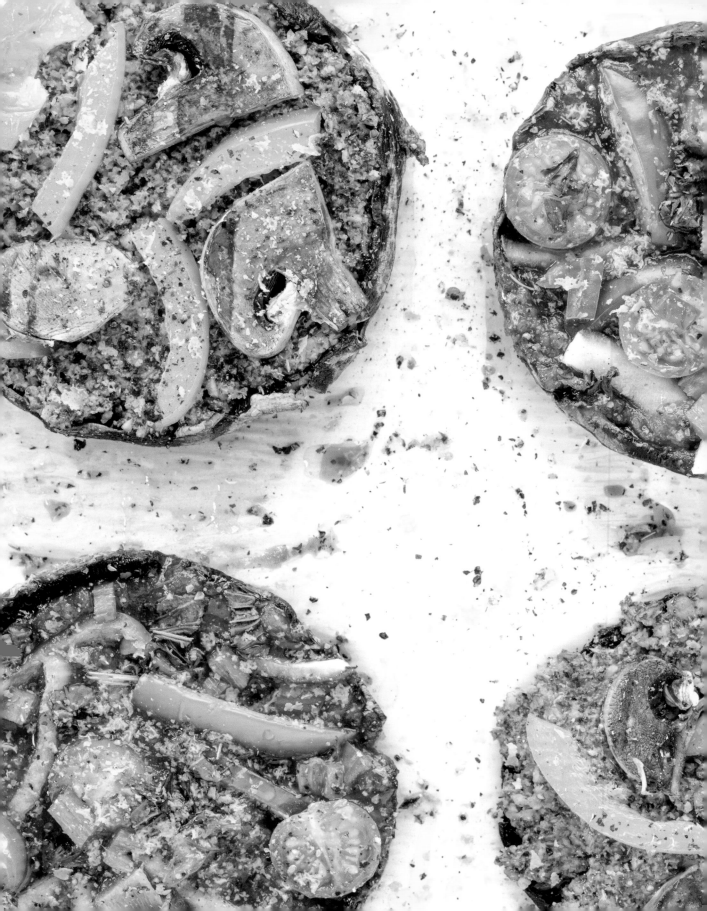

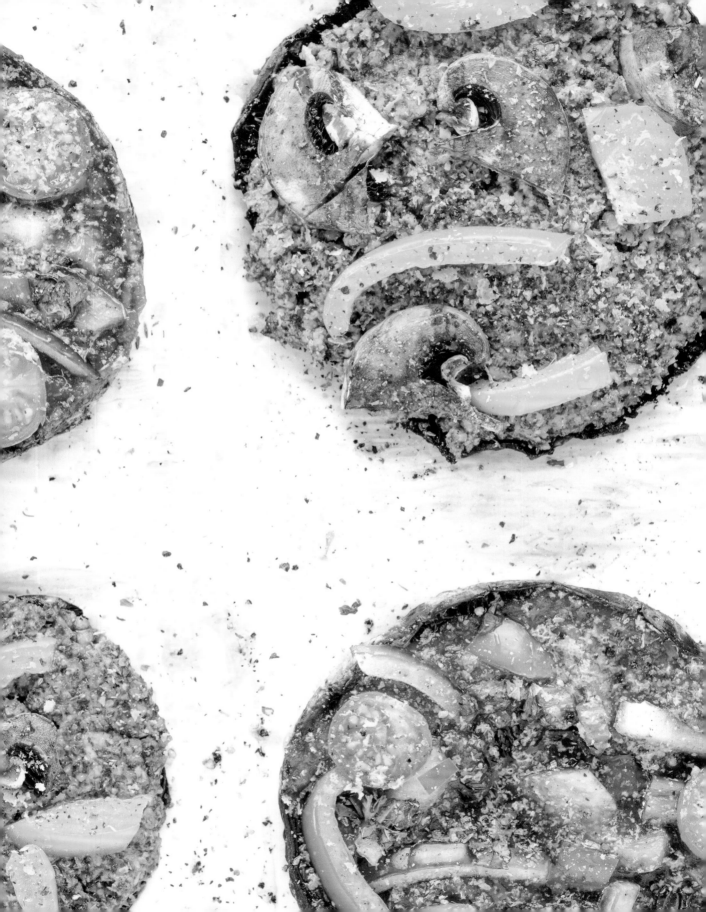

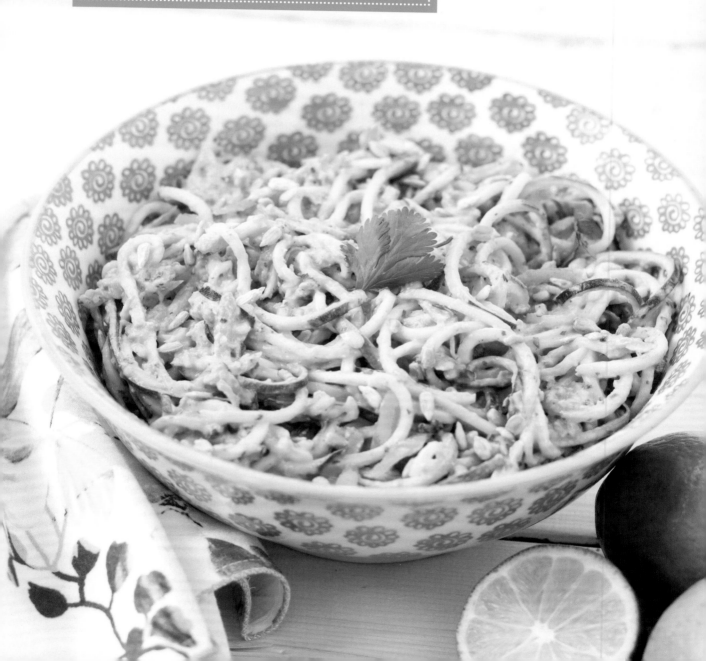

Zucchini Noodles with Avocado Cream Sauce

This is the definition of healthy fast food—totally raw, no-bake, yummy and filling zucchini noodles. People always go nuts for this when I post it on Instagram, and for good reason! The avocado cream sauce will make you totally forget that dairy sauce even existed. You can easily double the sauce if you're using larger zucchini.

Serves 2 as a main or 4 as a side dish

 Vegan   **Gluten-free**   **Dairy-free** **SF** **Sugar-free**

3 small zucchini

3 carrots

Garnishes: 1 tbsp (15 mL) raw sunflower seeds; 2 tbsp (30 mL) chopped fresh cilantro

Avocado Cream Sauce

1 large avocado, peeled and pitted

1 to 2 garlic cloves, crushed

1/2 cup (125 mL) loosely packed fresh cilantro

1/4 cup (60 mL) raw sunflower seeds

1/4 cup (60 mL) lime juice

1/4 cup (60 mL) extra-virgin olive oil

1/2 tsp (2 mL) cayenne pepper

Sea salt and pepper to taste

Spiralize zucchini and carrots. As the vegetables are being spiralized, use a pair of scissors to cut them every 5 inches (13 cm) or so to prevent the noodles from being too long and more difficult to eat. Set aside in a large bowl.

To make the avocado cream sauce, place all ingredients in a food processor or blender. Blend until creamy.

Combine sauce with spiralized zucchini and carrots. Garnish with sunflower seeds and cilantro.

Walker's Chicken with Fennel, Orange and Mint

My husband, Walker, is a great cook. Both his parents love good food, and lucky for me, they passed their passion on to him. Now I get to benefit from it! A perfect example is this absolutely delicious dish. The combination of fennel, orange and mint will delight your taste buds and you'll be going back for seconds—guaranteed. If you don't use all the orange chutney sauce, save it for a zesty addition to another dish.

Makes 2 servings

 Gluten-free Dairy-free 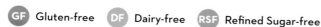 Refined Sugar-free

1 organic orange, unpeeled

2 tbsp (30 mL) liquid honey

2 tbsp (30 mL) white wine vinegar

2 boneless, skinless chicken breasts

Sea salt and black pepper

1 fennel bulb, thinly sliced

2 cups (500 mL) arugula

2 tbsp (30 mL) chopped fresh mint

2 tsp (10 mL) thinly sliced hot chili pepper

1 garlic clove, minced

1/2 cup (125 mL) extra-virgin olive oil

Cut ends off orange, slice into thin wedges and place in a medium saucepan. Add honey, vinegar and enough water to cover the orange wedges. Bring to a boil, reduce heat and simmer for 30 minutes to 1 hour, until you are left with 3 tbsp (45 mL) of syrup. Keep checking to make sure the water doesn't simmer away. If the liquid is getting too low, add a little more water. Scrape the contents into a food processor and blend until a chutney consistency. Transfer sauce to a medium bowl and set aside.

Heat a grill to medium-high. Season chicken with sea salt and pepper. Grill, turning once or twice, for 15 to 20 minutes or until there is no more pink inside the chicken or bake at 350°F (180°C) for 25 minutes.

Meanwhile, in a medium bowl, combine fennel with arugula, mint, chili peppers, garlic and 1/4 cup (60 mL) of the olive oil. Season with sea salt and pepper, then toss well.

Slice chicken into medium strips and mix with desired amount of orange chutney sauce. Add chicken to salad and toss. Add remaining 1/4 cup (60 mL) extra-virgin olive oil and season with sea salt and pepper.

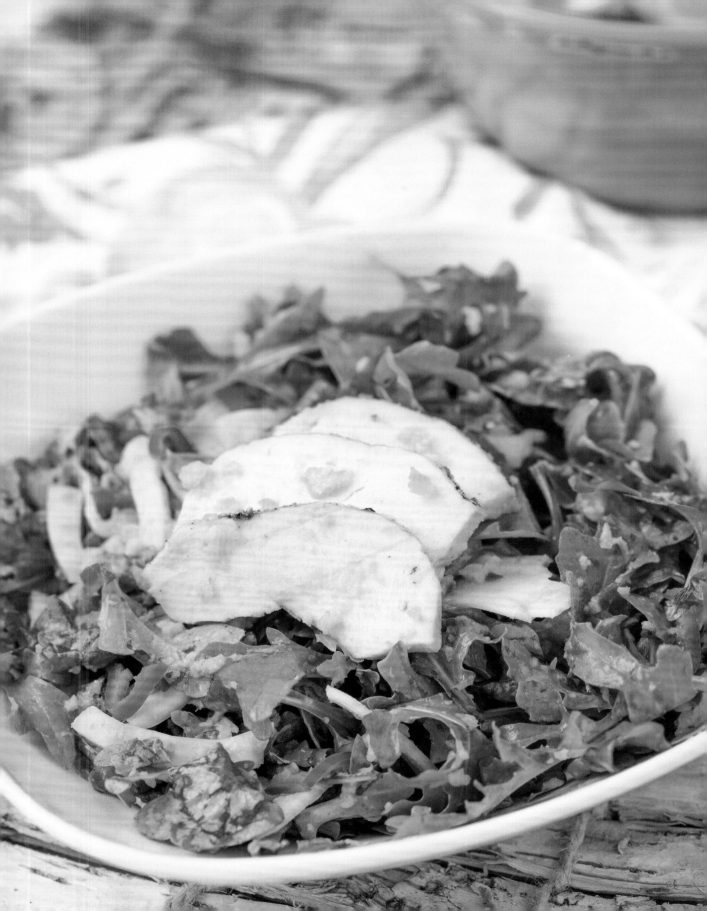

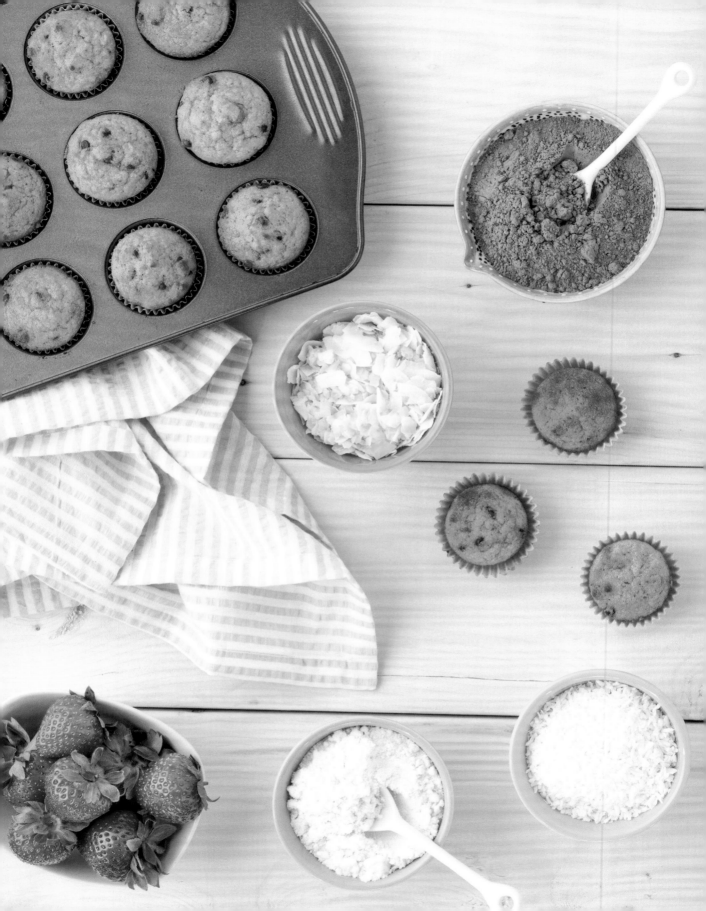

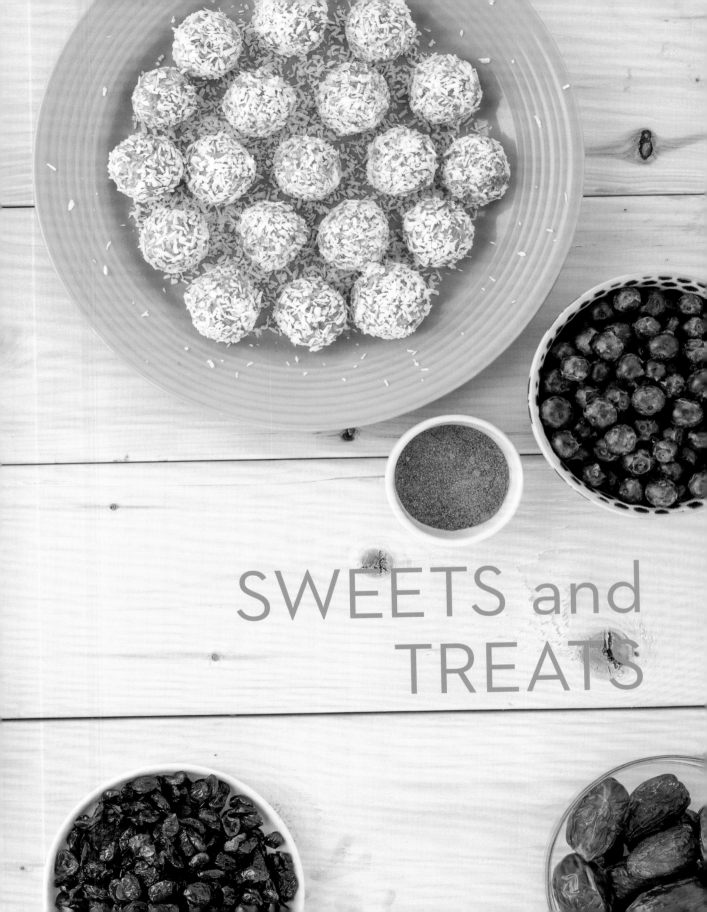

SWEETS and
TREATS

Pumpkin Chocolate Chip Mini Muffins

The regular-size version of these muffins is a *Joyous Health* blog reader favourite. I've revamped them a bit by making them in mini muffin tins. Perfect as a dessert or as a quick snack! You can always leave out the chocolate chips, if you prefer.

Makes 30 to 35 mini muffins

 Vegetarian   **Gluten-free**   **Dairy-free**   **Refined Sugar-free**

½ cup (125 mL) coconut flour

2½ tsp (12 mL) pumpkin pie spice (see tip)

2 tsp (10 mL) baking powder

¼ tsp (1 mL) fine sea salt

6 eggs

⅔ cup (150 mL) pumpkin purée

½ cup (125 mL) real maple syrup

½ cup (125 mL) coconut oil, melted

2 tsp (10 mL) pure vanilla extract

½ cup (125 mL) mini chocolate chips

Preheat oven to 350°F (180°C). Line a mini muffin pan with paper liners.

In a large bowl, whisk together coconut flour, pumpkin pie spice, baking powder and sea salt. In a separate bowl, whisk eggs, then whisk in pumpkin purée, maple syrup, coconut oil and vanilla. Add wet ingredients to dry ingredients and stir just until combined. Do not overmix. Fold in chocolate chips.

Spoon batter into mini muffin cups. Bake for 18 minutes or until a fork inserted into the middle of a muffin comes out clean. Turn out onto racks to cool.

> ## *Joyous Tip*
> • • •
> Coconut flour is a highly absorbent flour and expands a lot. This is why the amount of flour in this recipe is so small.
> If you want to make your own pumpkin pie spice, combine 1½ tsp (7 mL) cinnamon, ½ tsp (2 mL) nutmeg, ¼ tsp (1 mL) ground ginger and ¼ tsp (1 mL) ground cloves.

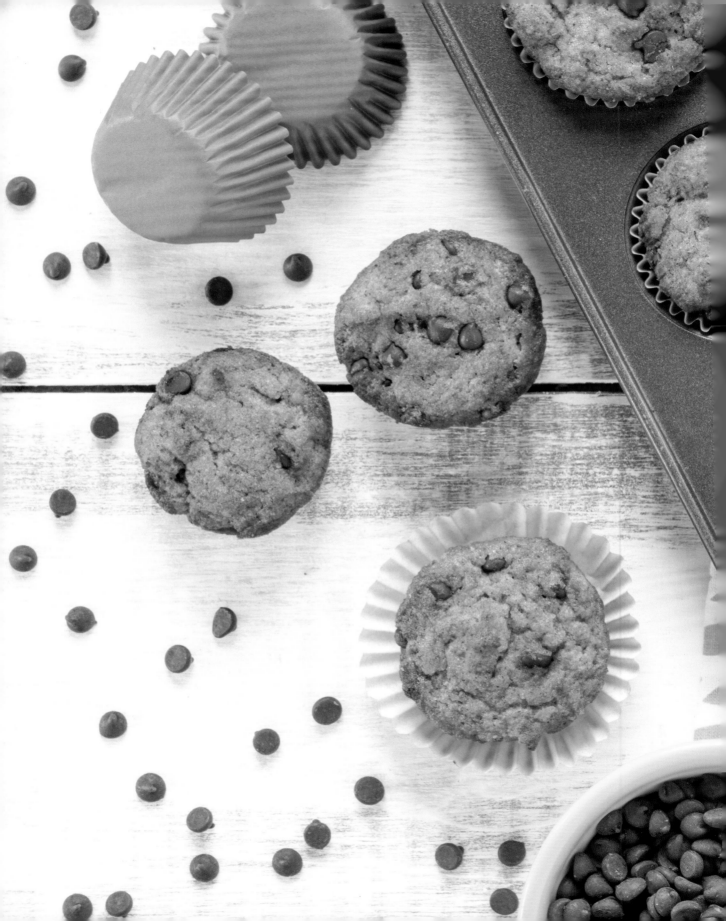

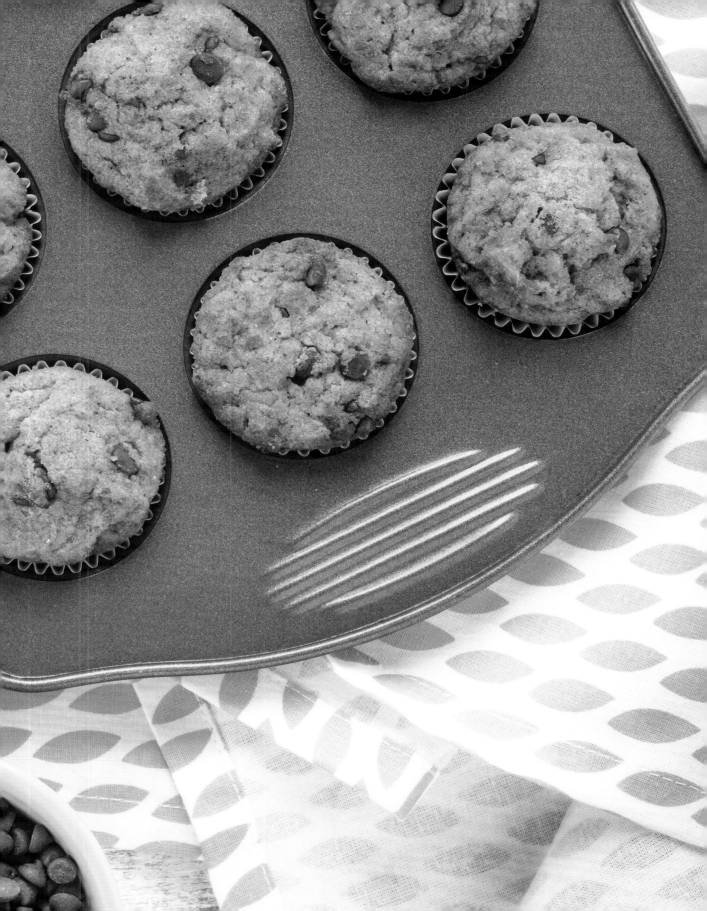

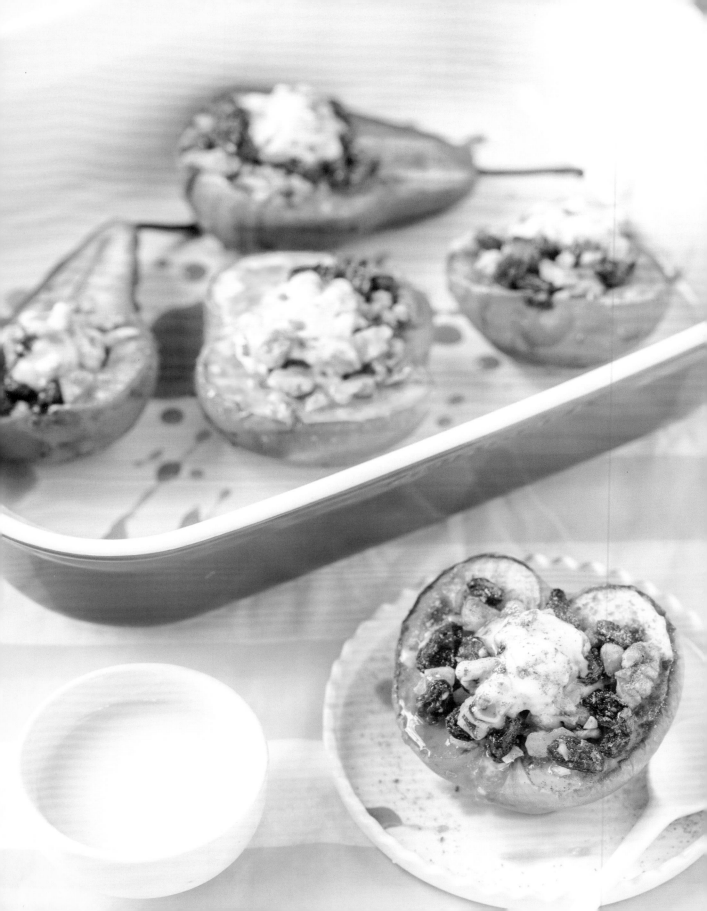

Ma McCarthy's Baked Apples and Pears with Coconut Butter

This was a healthy sweet treat my brother and I had as kids, especially in the fall when apples are in season. Coconut butter wasn't available back then, but it's a welcome addition today because it lends the perfect sweetness and texture to this wonderful recipe. Use an apple that holds its shape when baked. I find Gala, Honeycrisp, Pink Lady, Fuji and Granny Smith apples all work well.

Makes 8 servings

 Vegan   **Gluten-free**   **Dairy-free**   **Refined Sugar-free**

1 cup (250 mL) raisins

1 cup (250 mL) finely chopped walnuts

1 tsp (5 mL) cinnamon

2 apples, unpeeled

2 pears, unpeeled

½ cup (125 mL) apple juice or filtered water

¼ cup (60 mL) coconut butter

2 tbsp (30 mL) dark real maple syrup (optional)

Preheat oven to 400°F (200°C).

In a medium bowl, stir together raisins, walnuts and cinnamon. Set aside.

Cut apples and pears in half and remove the cores. In a shallow baking dish, arrange apples and pears cut side up. Pour enough apple juice over fruit to come ½ inch (1 cm) up the side of the pan. Spoon raisin-walnut mixture into the fruit cavities. Cover dish with a lid or foil and bake for 30 minutes or until soft.

Once fruit is cooked, place coconut butter in a small pot and warm it over the lowest heat until it becomes creamy. (It will not melt the way coconut oil does.) Be sure not to burn it.

Serve apples and pears topped with warmed coconut butter and drizzled with maple syrup if you like.

Joyous Tip

• • •

Apples are a detox superfood because they are a rich source of fibre that keeps you fuller longer, balances blood sugar and feeds good bacteria in your gut. Leave the skin on the apples and pears because this is where most of the nutrients are found, including the fibre and antioxidants.

Baked Brown Rice Pudding

Rice pudding has always been a favourite dessert of mine. I gave this traditional recipe a joyous makeover by using brown rice and whole foods to give it a naturally sweet taste. This is one of my go-to comfort recipes. You won't miss the white rice, refined sugar version at all.

Makes 6 servings

 Vegan　 **Gluten-free**　 **Dairy-free**　**SF** **Sugar-free**

1¼ cups (300 mL) brown rice

2½ cups (625 mL) filtered water

1 cup (250 mL) Medjool dates, pitted

2 medium bananas

1½ cups (375 mL) unsweetened almond milk

2 tsp (10 mL) pure vanilla extract

1 tsp (5 mL) cinnamon

¾ tsp (4 mL) ground ginger

¼ tsp (1 mL) ground cardamom

½ cup (125 mL) toasted unsweetened, unsulphured coconut flakes (optional)

¼ cup (60 mL) dried cranberries (optional)

Combine rice and water in a medium pot. Bring to a boil, then reduce heat, cover and simmer for 40 minutes or until rice is tender. Drain, then transfer to a large bowl.

Soak dates in warm water to cover for 30 minutes.

Meanwhile, preheat oven to 350°F (180°C). Grease a 9-inch (2.5 L) square baking dish.

Drain dates. In a blender or food processor, combine dates, bananas, almond milk, vanilla, cinnamon, ginger and cardamom. Blend until smooth. Stir date mixture into rice, then pour rice mixture into the baking dish.

Bake for 30 minutes. Let cool for a few minutes before spooning into serving bowls. Top with toasted coconut and cranberries, if desired.

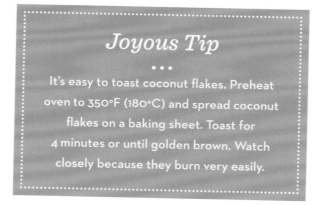

Joyous Tip

• • •

It's easy to toast coconut flakes. Preheat oven to 350°F (180°C) and spread coconut flakes on a baking sheet. Toast for 4 minutes or until golden brown. Watch closely because they burn very easily.

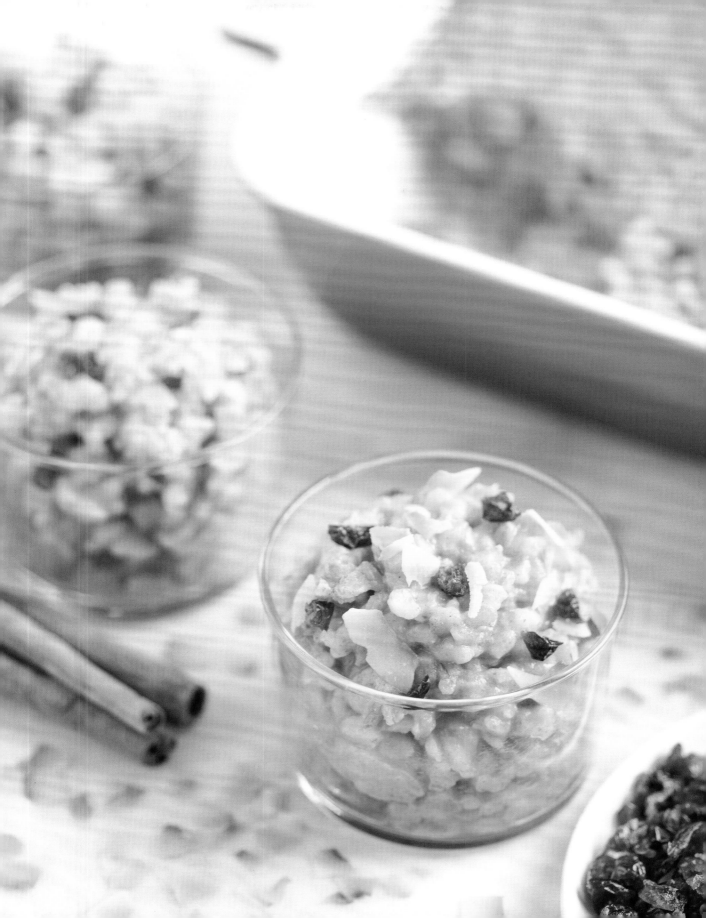

Chocolate Chia Mousse

This recipe is always a crowd-pleaser because who doesn't love chocolate mousse? You'll love the creamy, silky texture minus the refined sugar that your typical store-bought pudding contains.

Makes 4 servings

 Vegan   Gluten-free   Dairy-free   Refined Sugar-free

4 Medjool dates, pitted

1 can (14 oz/400 mL) full-fat coconut milk

½ cup (125 mL) raw cacao powder

¼ cup (60 mL) chia seeds

¼ cup (60 mL) real maple syrup

Garnishes

½ cup (125 mL) thinly sliced fresh strawberries

2 tbsp (10 mL) raw cacao nibs

2 tbsp (10 mL) unsweetened, unsulphured coconut flakes

Soak dates in water to cover for 2 hours. Drain.

In a high-speed blender or food processor, place dates, coconut milk, cacao powder, chia seeds and maple syrup. Blend until fully combined. Pour pudding into individual serving bowls. Cover and refrigerate for at least 4 hours.

Garnish with fresh strawberries, cacao nibs and coconut flakes.

> *Joyous Tip*
>
> • • •
>
> Because canned coconut milk is richer in fat than homemade, after the mousse has thickened in the fridge feel free to thin out the consistency by adding a little more coconut milk if desired. If the mousse is not thick enough, add more chia seeds.
> For a step-by-step video of this recipe, visit joyoushealth.com/chocolatemousse.

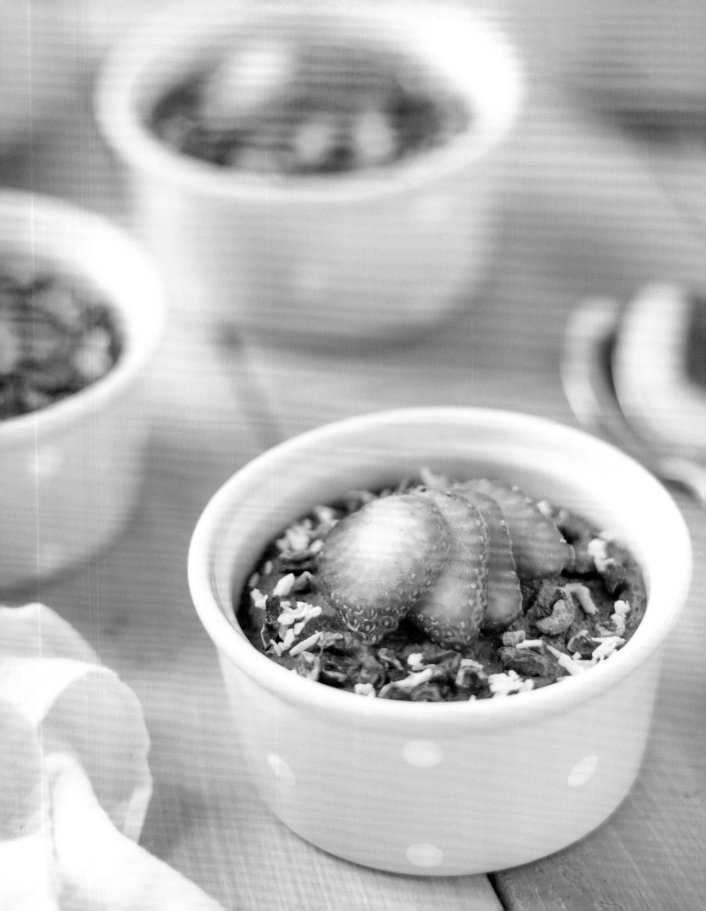

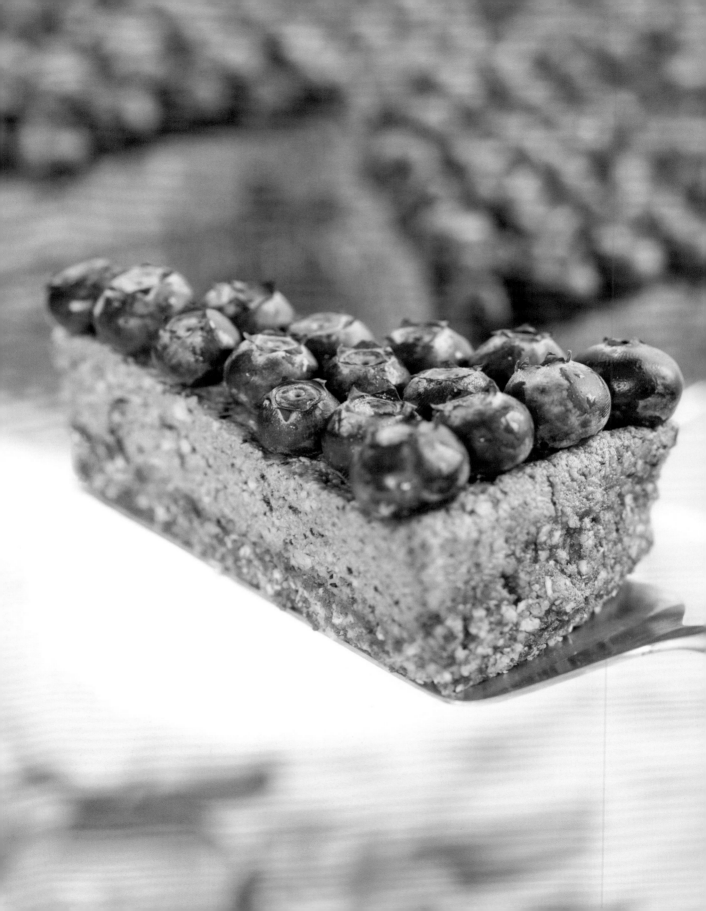

Rawkin' Blueberry "Cheezecake"

Every time I make this "cheezecake" for a dinner party, I secretly hope there will be at least one slice left that I can enjoy the next day. It is creamy, incredibly flavourful and totally guilt-free. You'll love how easy it is to make because it's no-bake.

Makes 8 to 10 servings

 V Vegetarian **GF** Gluten-free **DF** Dairy-free **RSF** Refined Sugar-free

Crust

10 to 12 soft Medjool dates, pitted

2 cups (500 mL) walnuts

¾ cup (175 mL) unsweetened, unsulphured shredded coconut

3 tbsp (45 mL) cinnamon

Filling

2 cups (500 mL) raw cashews

1¼ cups (300 mL) fresh or thawed frozen blueberries (see tip)

¼ cup (60 mL) coconut oil

1 tsp (5 mL) pure vanilla extract

¼ cup (60 mL) liquid honey or real maple syrup (optional)

1 pint (500 mL) fresh blueberries

Soak cashews for the filling in water to cover for at least 4 hours or overnight. Drain and set aside.

To make the crust, in a food processor or high-speed blender, place dates, walnuts, coconut and cinnamon. Process until the mixture is smoother but still a bit crumbly. Press crust mixture into the bottom and partway up the sides of a 9-inch (23 cm) springform pan. Place in the freezer to chill while you prepare the filling.

To make the filling, in the cleaned food processor or blender, combine cashews, 1¼ cups (300 mL) blueberries, coconut oil and vanilla. Blend until smooth. Taste, and add honey if the filling is too tart. Pour the filling into the chilled crust. Cover and freeze until solid, at least 4 hours. Transfer to the fridge and let thaw for an hour before serving. Serve topped with fresh blueberries.

> ## *Joyous Tip*
> • • •
> If you're using frozen blueberries, thaw them first and drain them. The thawed berries will make the filling a bit wetter, so you may need to use more cashews to compensate. You can use any size pan. Just remember that the smaller the pan, the thicker the crust, and the larger the pan, the thinner the crust.

No-Bake Carrot Cake Squares with Lemon Icing

Carrot cake is my all-time favourite dessert. However, the traditional recipe is not detox friendly. These delicious squares have all the flavour but none of the guilt. I highly recommend you enjoy them with a Matcha Coconut Milk Latte on page 158.

Makes 8 squares

 Vegetarian   Gluten-free   Dairy-free   Refined Sugar-free

Carrot Cake

12 Medjool dates, pitted

3 medium carrots, cut into chunks

1 1/2 cups (375 mL) walnuts

1 cup (250 mL) unsweetened, unsulphured shredded coconut

1/2 cup (125 mL) shelled hemp seeds or vanilla plant-based protein powder

1/2 cup (125 mL) liquid honey

2 tsp (10 mL) pure vanilla extract (if not using vanilla protein powder)

2 tsp (10 mL) cinnamon

1 tsp (5 mL) nutmeg

1/2 tsp (2 mL) ground cloves

Lemon Icing

1/2 cup (125 mL) coconut butter, room temperature

1/4 cup (60 mL) liquid honey

1 tsp (5 mL) pure vanilla extract

1/2 tsp (2 mL) lemon zest

2 tbsp (30 mL) unsweetened almond milk (optional)

To make the cake, place all ingredients in a food processor and blend until almost smooth. You may need to do this in two batches. Press mixture into an 8-inch (2 L) square cake pan. Chill in fridge for 1 to 2 hours.

Meanwhile, to make the icing, in the cleaned food processor, combine the coconut butter, honey, vanilla and lemon zest. Blend until creamy. Add almond milk if you want a thinner consistency.

Spread icing evenly on top of chilled cake. Refrigerate or freeze until ready to enjoy.

> ## Joyous Tip
> • • •
> The cake will be easier to cut if you freeze it. Just let it sit for a few minutes once you remove it from the freezer, otherwise the icing will be crumbly when you cut it.

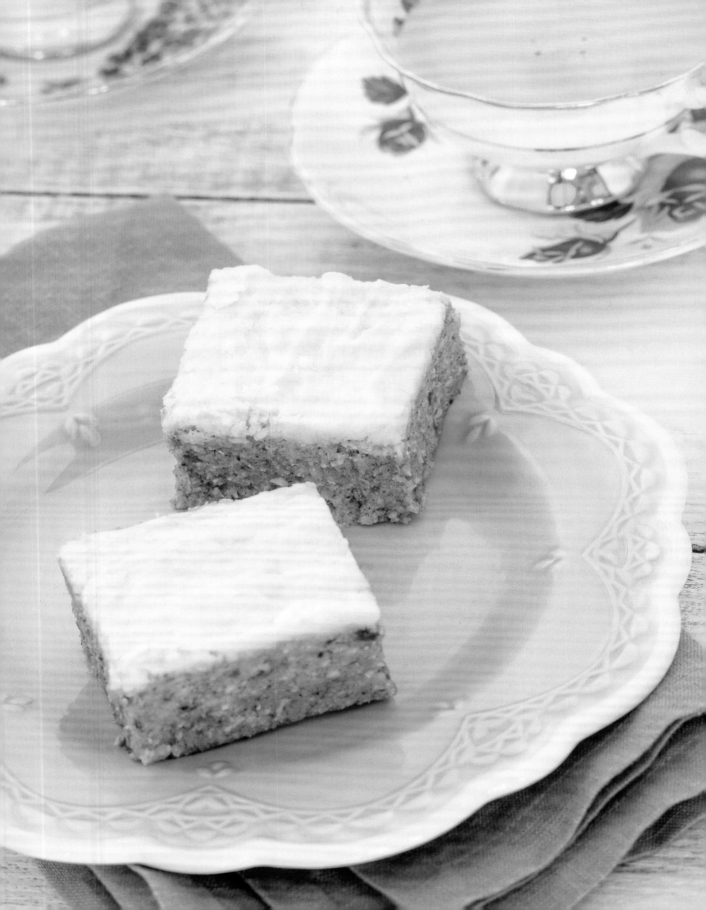

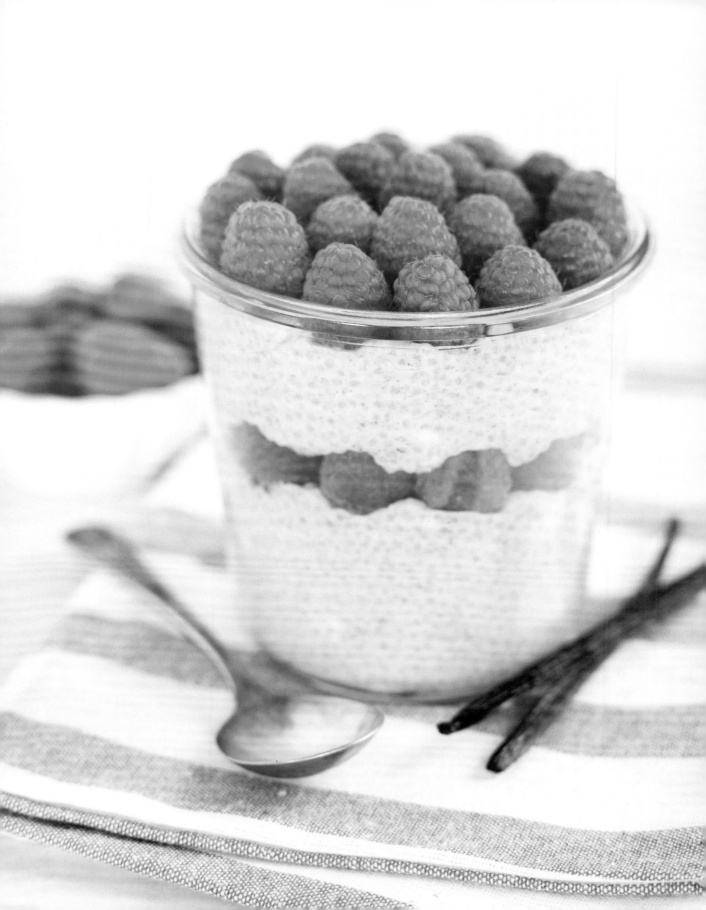

Raspberry Vanilla Bean Chia Pudding

Your taste buds will never know this recipe is healthy (nor will anyone you make it for) because it is so incredibly yummy and creamy.

Makes 4 to 6 servings

 Vegan **Gluten-free** **Dairy-free** **Refined Sugar-free**

1 can (14 oz/400 mL) full-fat coconut milk

½ cup (125 mL) filtered water

⅓ cup (75 mL) chia seeds

2 tbsp (30 mL) real maple syrup

½ tsp (2 mL) vanilla powder (or 1 tsp/5 mL pure vanilla extract)

1 pint (500 mL) fresh raspberries

1 tsp (5 mL) cinnamon

In a medium bowl, combine coconut milk, water, chia seeds, maple syrup and vanilla. Stir well. Cover and refrigerate for at least 4 hours.

Serve with fresh raspberries and a sprinkle of cinnamon on top.

> ## Joyous Tip
> • • •
> If you are using canned coconut milk, it will be much thicker than homemade, so you may want to stir a little more coconut milk into your pudding after it has chilled.

Apple Pie Bites

Growing up, Sunday evenings often meant a family dinner with both of my grandmas. More often than not, my mom would either bake apple crisp or buy an apple pie from the local farmers' market. Those memories inspired me to create these apple pie bites. Enjoy 1 or 2 as a snack or dessert.

Makes 18 to 20 balls

 Vegan   Gluten-free   Dairy-free   Refined Sugar-free

¾ cup (175 mL) unsweetened, unsulphured shredded coconut

6 Medjool dates, pitted

1 apple (unpeeled if organic), cored and chopped into large chunks

1 cup (250 mL) cashews or walnuts

¼ cup (60 mL) chia seeds

¼ cup (60 mL) vanilla or unflavoured plant-based protein powder (or ¼ cup/60 mL quinoa flour or brown rice flour)

2 tbsp (30 mL) cinnamon

½ tsp (2 mL) nutmeg

1 tbsp (15 mL) fresh lemon juice

1 tsp (5 mL) pure vanilla extract (if not using vanilla protein powder)

Pinch of sea salt

Reserve ¼ cup (60 mL) shredded coconut in a shallow dish for rolling.

Place remaining ingredients in a food processor and process until fully combined. The mixture will be soft and delicate, but it will harden up once chilled. If it's too wet to roll into balls, add ¼ cup (60 mL) more cashews or walnuts and blend again. Form mixture into 1-inch (2.5 cm) balls and roll in reserved shredded coconut, coating balls completely.

Arrange balls on a baking sheet and refrigerate or freeze for a few hours or overnight. To store, keep chilled, or freeze in an airtight container for a few months (though I guarantee they won't last that long).

Mango Lassi Pudding

Next time you have a perfectly ripe mango, resist the temptation to eat it immediately, and instead make this mousse. It's a guilt-free and detoxifying sweet treat you'll love.

Makes 4 servings

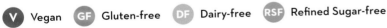 **V** Vegan **GF** Gluten-free **DF** Dairy-free **RSF** Refined Sugar-free

1 ²/₃ cups (400 mL) unsweetened rice or almond milk

1 cup (250 mL) chopped fresh or thawed frozen mango

¹/₄ cup (60 mL) chia seeds

1 tsp (5 mL) pure vanilla extract

¹/₂ tsp (2 mL) ground cardamom

Place all ingredients in a high-speed blender or food processor. Blend until fully combined. Pour pudding into individual serving bowls or one large bowl. Cover and refrigerate for at least 4 hours.

Chocolate Ice Pops

When the heat of the summer hits, these creamy rich ice pops will cool you off. They remind me of the sugar-filled Fudgsicles I used to eat as a kid, but they're way healthier!

Makes about 4 ice pops, depending on size of ice-pop mould

 Vegan   Gluten-free   Dairy-free **RSF** Refined Sugar-free

1 can (14 oz/400 mL) full-fat coconut milk
¼ cup (60 mL) raw cacao powder
2 to 3 tbsp (30 to 45 mL) real maple syrup
2 tbsp (30 mL) mini dairy-free chocolate chips

Place all ingredients except chocolate chips in a food processor or blender and whirl until fully combined. Pour into ice-pop moulds, toss in a few chocolate chips and freeze until mixture starts to solidify, a couple of hours. Insert sticks, then freeze completely.

Joyous Tip

• • •

Instead of maple syrup, you can sweeten the ice pops with 2 pitted Medjool dates, 1 banana or 10 drops liquid stevia. I suggest you taste the blended mixture and decide if you want a sweeter taste. Sometimes pure raw cacao powder can have a slightly bitter aftertaste.

Strawberry Mylkshake

This mylkshake is detox friendly because it is free of dairy. But don't worry, you won't miss the milk because it's just as delicious.

Makes 1 to 2 servings

 Vegan Gluten-free Dairy-free Refined Sugar-free

1 frozen banana

1 cup (250 mL) fresh or frozen strawberries

2 tbsp (30 mL) coconut butter

¼ cup (60 mL) shelled hemp seeds

1 cup (250 mL) Nutty Milk (page 148)

1 tbsp (15 mL) chia seeds

Garnishes: 1 tbsp (15 mL) unsweetened, unsulphured coconut flakes; 1 tbsp (15 mL) cacao nibs

Place all ingredients except garnishes in a blender and whirl until smooth and creamy. For a little crunch, garnish with coconut flakes and cacao nibs.

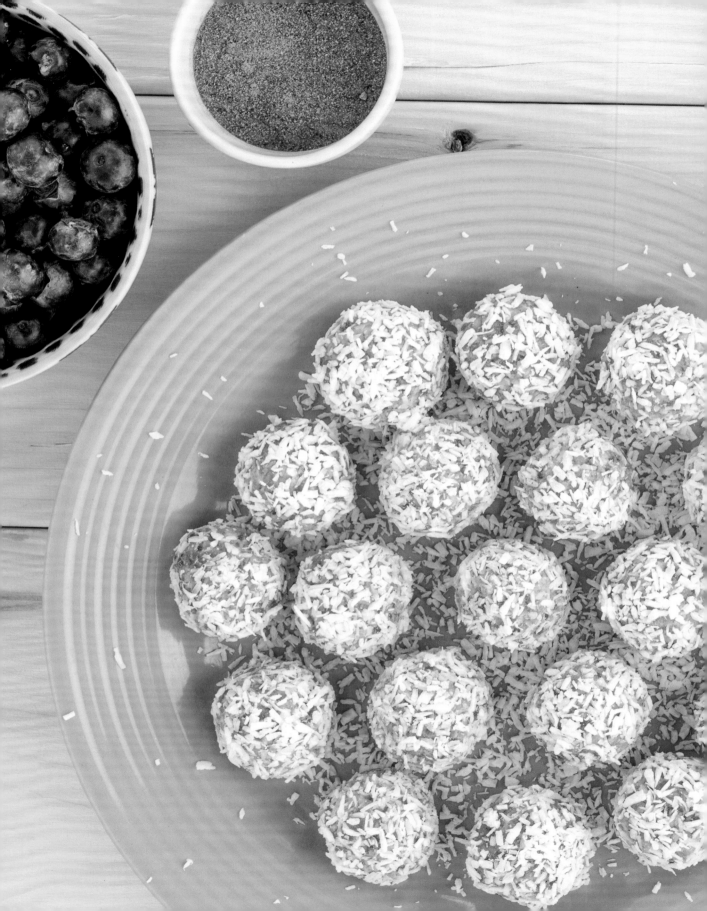

Lemon Ginger Snowballs

These delicious no-bake snowballs burst with bright flavours from the lemon and ginger. A perfect detox-friendly treat to satisfy your sweet tooth and balance your blood sugar.

Makes 18 to 20 balls

 Vegetarian   **Gluten-free**   **Dairy-free**   **Refined Sugar-free**

1³⁄₄ cups (425 mL) unsweetened, unsulphured coconut flakes

¹⁄₄ cup (60 mL) lemon juice

¹⁄₄ cup (60 mL) coconut oil, room temperature

¹⁄₄ cup (60 mL) liquid honey

1 tbsp (15 mL) grated fresh ginger

Reserve ¼ cup (60 mL) of the coconut flakes in a shallow dish for rolling.

Place remaining ingredients in a food processor and blend until smooth. Roll into 1½-inch (4 cm) balls and then roll in reserved coconut flakes. Arrange on a baking sheet and freeze for at least 4 hours. Keep frozen. Thaw for 10 minutes before serving.

> ## *Joyous Tip*
> • • •
> Buy unpasteurized honey. It is richer in nutrients such as B vitamins, good bacteria, enzymes and amino acids. Want to make this vegan? Use maple syrup in place of the honey.

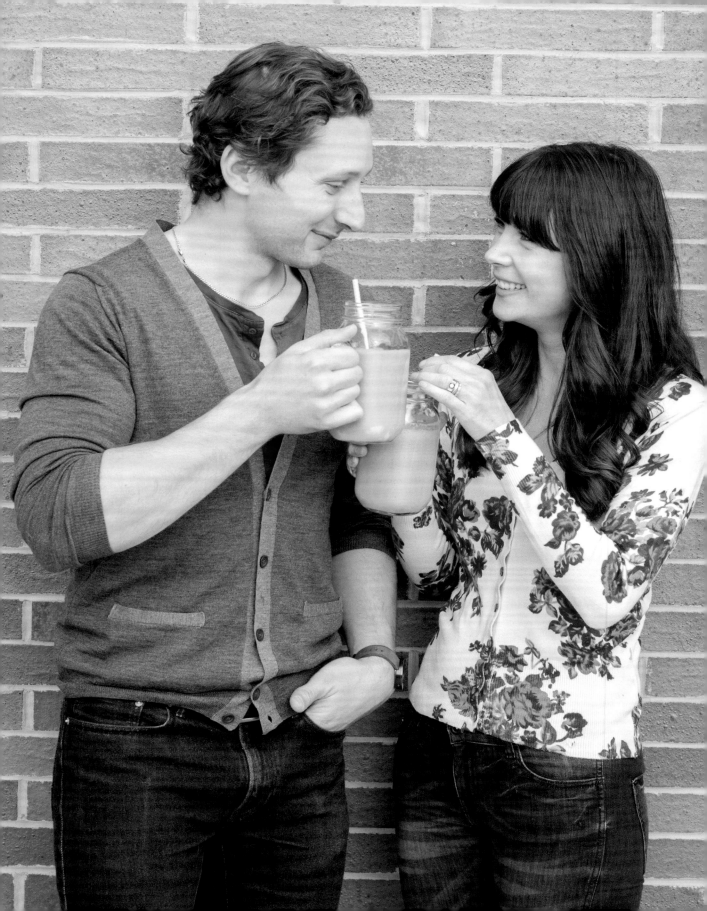

*Wishing you joyous health
today and always!*

ACKNOWLEDGMENTS

Walker—This book is dedicated to you, the love of my life, incredible father to our sweet bean, Vienna, business partner, best friend and real food lover. For the amazing man who always knows how to make me laugh, gives the best hugs, can whip up an incredible meal without ever using a recipe and is the most dependable man I know—my husband, Walker Jordan—to infinity and beyond, thank you!

My sweet bean, Vienna—We wrote this entire book together. The nine plus months that I was pregnant with you, your spirit was always cheering me on with your pokes, dance moves and nuzzles. I can't wait to create magic with you in the kitchen and get messy!

Mom a.k.a. Ma McCarthy—You're my living guardian angel and the sweetest, most thoughtful woman I know. Thank you for being the first to read *Joyous Detox* with your eagle eye and for all your endless hours helping to convert my recipes to metric.

Dad—You're an inspiration to me. You are a beaming ray of positivity, love and strength. Thank you for teaching me how to have a sense of humour even in the tough times.

Carol—My design goddess of all things Joyous Health and food stylist for this book. Thank you for your creative brilliance and sweet sunshiny personality. You are always a joy to work with.

Chris—My incredibly talented and very joyful photographer. You've been an absolute pleasure to work with on *Joyous Detox* and other projects. Thank you for always being so flexible, easy to work with and so much fun!

Lynsey—My right-hand lady when we were shooting all the recipes for this book. I was just entering my third trimester of pregnancy and making over sixty recipes from scratch for the photoshoot. I couldn't have done it without you by my side in the kitchen!

Mark a.k.a. benchy—My long-time dear friend. Thank you for encouraging me to pursue my passion studying at the Institute of Holistic Nutrition and opening my eyes to the world of organic food many years ago.

Kate—My resident (and favourite) nutrient nerd/editing guru at Joyous Health. Thank you for your endless hours reviewing my manuscript.

Shaun—My official copy editor. Thank you for your razor-sharp editing skills.

Laura—A full-time teacher and mama to two beautiful children. Thank you for being my official recipe tester. Your passion and enthusiasm for organic, whole food is inspiring.

Andrea—My editor. It has been an absolute pleasure working with you, and I'm so grateful for the opportunity to create this book. Thank you to the entire team at Penguin Random House Canada for making this book possible.

Rick—My literary agent. Thank you for always looking out for my best interests professionally. You're fierce!

Last but certainly not least, to all the *Joyous Health* readers and social media community who inspire me with your health transformations, Instagram food photos and stories—thank you for your support and love over the years.

Joyous Affirmation

I am grateful for this opportunity to take good care of myself because I am positively glowing and my health is on the right track.

INDEX

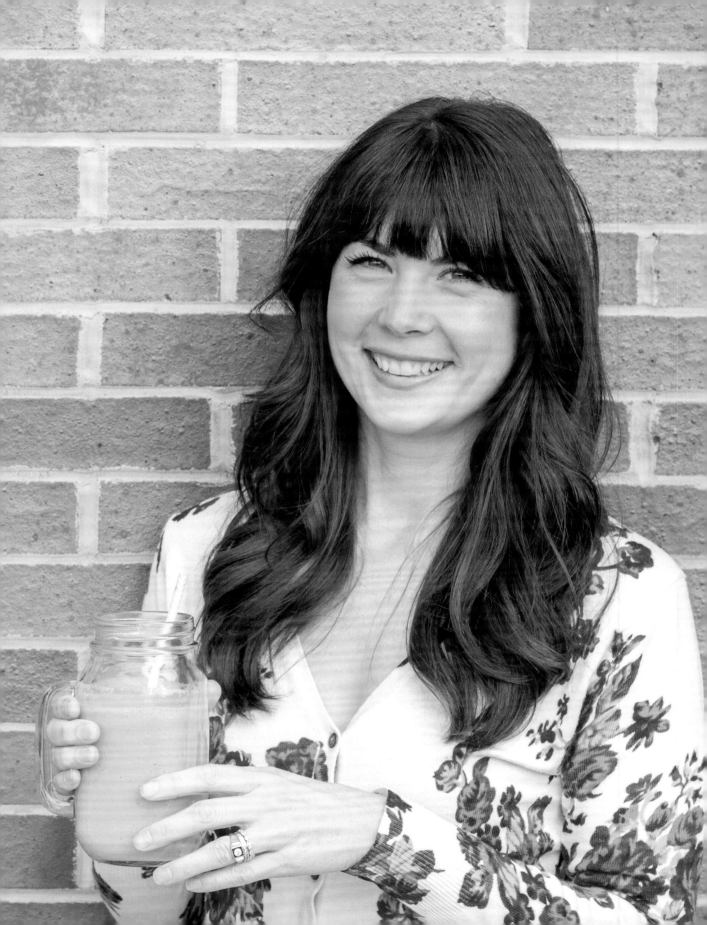

ABOUT JOY McCARTHY

Joy McCarthy, CNP, is the bestselling author of *Joyous Health: Eat and Live Well Without Dieting* and the vibrant nutritionist behind the healthy living blog JoyousHealth.com, whose expertise has helped people around the world achieve their wellness goals. She is a noted international wellness speaker and a faculty member at the Institute of Holistic Nutrition.

Her infectious energy and passion for whole foods has led to her being featured as a nutrition expert in hundreds of media outlets, including television, radio, print and online, among them Global TV's *Morning Show*, CNN, CBC, CTV News, *The Globe and Mail*, *Chatelaine*, *Fashion* and *Elle Canada*.

She is the founder of Eat Well Feel Well, Toronto's longest-running holistic nutrition and yoga program. Joy is fiercely committed to clean beauty products and has a line of toxin-free natural body care products.

Joy is a graduate (with honours) of the Institute of Holistic Nutrition (IHN), has a certification in Clinical Detoxification from IHN, is a professional member of the International Organization of Nutritional Consultants and is a Registered Orthomolecular Health Practitioner.

Joy lives in Toronto with her husband, Walker, their daughter, Vienna, and their two cats, Miss Nellers and Theo.

Joyous Affirmation

I am the architect of my well-being.
I build its foundation with every choice I make.